THE ART OF FEEDING CHILDREN WELL

D0103998

OTHER BOOKS BY DR. MICHAEL A. WEINER

Earth Medicine—Earth Food
Plant a Tree
Man's Useful Plants
Homeopathic Medicine
In Search of the Durian
Nutritional Ethnomedicine in Fiji
Weiner's Herbal
The Way of the Skeptical Nutritionist

The Art of Feeding Children Well

by Dr. Michael A. Weiner

and Kathleen Goss

WARNER BOOKS

A Warner Communications Company

Copyright © 1982 by Michael A. Weiner

All rights reserved.

Warner Books, Inc., 75 Rockefeller Plaza, New York, N. Y. 10019

W A Warner Communications Company

Printed in the United States of America

First Printing: January 1982

10 9 8 7 6 5 4 3 2 1

Book design by H. Roberts Design

Cover design by The New Studio

Grateful acknowledgment is made for permission to reprint copyrighted material:

From I. N. Kugelmass, *The Newer Nutrition in Pediatric Practice,* Lippincott, 1940. Reprinted by permission of Lippincott/Harper & Row.

From the Weimar Kitchen. Reprinted by permission of the Weimar Institute, Weimar, CA.

Library of Congress Cataloging in Publication Data

Weiner, Michael A.
    The art of feeding children well.

    Bibliography: p.
    Includes index.
    1. Children—Nutrition.   2.   Diet therapy for
    children.   I.   Goss, Kathleen.   II.   Title.
    RJ206.W37   613.2′088054   81-3044
    ISBN 0-446-97890-6 (U.S.A.) AACR2
    ISBN 0-446-37086-X (Canada)

ATTENTION: SCHOOLS AND CORPORATIONS

WARNER books are available at quantity discounts with bulk purchase for educational, business, or sales promotional use. For information, please write to: SPECIAL SALES DEPARTMENT, WARNER BOOKS, 75 ROCKEFELLER PLAZA, NEW YORK, N.Y. 10019.

ARE THERE WARNER BOOKS
YOU WANT BUT CANNOT FIND IN YOUR LOCAL STORES?

You can get any WARNER BOOKS title in print. Simply send title and retail price, plus 50¢ per order and 50¢ per copy to cover mailing and handling costs for each book desired. New York State and California residents add applicable sales tax. Enclose check or money order only, no cash please, to: WARNER BOOKS, P.O. BOX 690, NEW YORK, N.Y. 10019. OR SEND FOR OUR COMPLETE CATALOGUE OF WARNER BOOKS.

PREFACE

Just as the undrawn sword is the mark of the best swordsman, so too is the best physician one who relies least on synthetic drugs to heal. As a nutritionist by training, I have not had to overcome an inherent bias in favor of prescription drugs; food has always seemed the best medicine to me, especially as a preventive practice.

There is a tendency today for once-drug-oriented physicians to proselytize about "nutrition" while recommending highly questionable glandular extracts (particularly the adrenal) and drug-size doses of vitamins and minerals. These new converts seem to forget that "nutrition" also means *food!* In my program of preventive dietetics, food is first, with *minor* vitamin and mineral supplementation as an adjunct.

In cases of minor illness, we recommend modified diets, in conjunction with herbal teas. For this purpose special diets for states of illness are included, such as the liquid diet, the soft diet, and the low-residue diet. These diets for disease states are designed for parents and pediatricians who are interested in overcoming the "flaw in medical education." Synthetic drugs, surgery, and the entire arsenal of space-age medicine *do* have a place in medical care, but should be reserved for severe or stubborn cases. If your pediatrician agrees that the symptoms are not alarming, the more natural nutritional approach should be your first course of action.

We do *not* believe in telling you what to eat or how to feed your children on a day-to-day, meal-to-meal basis. That just takes the spontaneity and pleasure out of life. To introduce you to some healthful alternatives to the usual daily dietary routine, however, we provide some meat-, sugar-, egg-, dairy-, and oil-free recipes in Book IV, "Receipes for Resisters." By using these dishes in conjunction with typical American protein foods such as meat, fish, and poultry, you and your family will be practicing the best preventive nutrition, without having to accept the imposition of a rigid diet regime—a "food fascism."

The time has come for medical practitioners to listen to their patients who increasingly "talk" nutritional prevention and therapy. Parents who have read much on the subject are often ahead of established medical thinking.

Nutritional science is still in its infancy and does not have *all* the answers to our many questions. What we *do* have is a set of coordinates through which we can draw a line, but by no means does this line represent the ultimate path to nutritional wisdom. Present and future research, analyzed in the context of more ancient dietary laws, can eventually lead us to as near perfect states of health as we are genetically capable of achieving.

CONTENTS

TABLES

BOOK I
Laying the Nutritional Groundwork

FEEDING FOR PREVENTION

CANCER A LEADING CAUSE OF CHILDREN'S DEATH

One of the most suppressed statistics is that more children under the age of fifteen die of cancer, including leukemia, than of any other cause aside from accidents. This alarming fact is reason for worry, but not despair, because there is now a trend away from a "magic bullet" approach to cancer toward the preventive concept of altering environmental factors associated with certain cancers.

CANCER IS MULTIFACTORIAL IN ORIGIN

Certainly food and diet are such environmental factors. To reduce the cancer risk we may adjust the diet of our children, eliminating additives, chemicals, and sucrose while increasing fruit and vegetable intake. Still the best-fed children contract cancer and other illnesses. Diet is important, but so is heredity. In those tragic cases in which the well-fed and well-cared-for child develops cancer, environmental causes other than food and drink may be involved. Pesticides, industrial contamination of air and water, are often cited, but the state of the parents' health prior to conception, and of the mother during gestation and nursing, may also be critical factors. Here is where preventive nutrition can play a major role in health assurance.

PEDIATRICIANS OFTEN UNINFORMED ABOUT NUTRITION

Parents often think that pediatricians know enough about child feeding to provide adequate guidance. Unfortunately, in my own experience with major metropolitan hospitals I have found that pediatricians often know *less* about proper diet during states of illness and for maintenance of health than do most educated parents! This is particularly surprising when you consider that pediatrics developed as a specialty because internists "did not know how to feed babies." In this sense pediatrics was a nutritionally induced specialty, according to Dr. Jan Van Eys, chairman of pediatrics at the M. D. Anderson Hospital, in Houston, Texas.

WEINER PROGRAM IS CENTRIST

My program of childhood feeding is not designed to tempt jaded appetites. Food technologists who offer children a thirty-first version of sugary breakfast foods and a hundred-and-first version of denatured pastry are creating for those parents and children who are selecting themselves out of the evolutionary process. By violating nature's laws and eating unnatural diets of fabricated foods, these unfortunate consumers greatly increase their risk of developing cancer, diabetes, heart disease, behavioral disorders, and other ailments of civilization. Our preventive program emphasizes a nonextremist diet and is balanced well beyond the four-food-group propaganda. The dietary principles of Book II herein, "The

Diet of Older Children," are designed for thoughtful parents, those with enough will to say no where a "no" is required and the sense to realize that nutrition can no longer be guided by the intuitive "eat as you want" notion that once seemed reasonable to uncritical minds. With the advent of food technology and the overwhelming influence of advertising, few of us are able to follow our true food instincts, even if by doing so we would eat what our bodies required for proper nutrition.

The subject of nutrition is now so splintered by dietary theorists as to be incomprehensible to even the highly educated parent. What we propose as a preventive diet is a centrist approach in which both animal and vegetable products are eaten. A rearrangement of the relative proportions of vegetables, fruits, nuts, fleshy and dairy products, accompanied by a definite but modest program of supplementation (to augment those nutrients in short supply in even the most superior Western diet), will improve the health of our children. Allergies, colds, low energy, crankiness, headaches, stomach upsets—all the complaints that trouble the average growing child (and his or her parents)—can be greatly reduced.

Food the Best Medicine

HOW TO FEED DURING ILLNESS OFTEN OVERLOOKED

Even the healthiest primitive warriors fell ill occasionally, as do our Tom Sawyers and Becky Thatchers. By knowing which foods to withhold and which to offer, as well as special herbal-tea recipes when illness occurs, you will have the option of aiding your child without total dependency on costly and often dangerous prescription drugs. These diets for illness are presented in Book III, "Natural Approaches for Natural Complaints." In a sense, diet is the primary form of drugless therapy we have at our disposal, and like the ancients who viewed food "as medicine" we too can learn to manipulate our menus, to make the normal days better and to minimize the number of days of illness.

RECOMMENDED DIETARY ALLOWANCES (RDAs): WHAT THEY MEAN

RDA NOT MEANT FOR INDIVIDUAL USE

The RDA (Recommended Dietary Allowance) for a given nutrient is based upon the *mean* quantity of that nutrient required by a total population. This means that half of us who eat less than this RDA might show *no* signs of deficiency, and half of us who eat more than this RDA may still show signs of deficiency. To allow for variable needs among individuals, the RDA for each nutrient is set at two standard deviations above the mean. What this means is that 98 percent of all healthy people in this population will have their needs for specific nutrients satisfied if they consume and absorb the RDA of each nutrient. Of course, some individuals do not need even these minimal RDAs, because their bodies can adapt to low nutrient levels. On the other hand, 2 percent of the population (over 4 million people!) will be deficient in some nutrients at RDA levels. The eminent biochemist Roger Williams estimates that *some* of us may need upwards of *15 times* more than the RDA of certain essential nutrients.

WHAT IS ABSORBED IS WHAT COUNTS

Even if the RDA for a given nutrient is the actual amount needed to maintain health in an "average" child or adult (see Appendix A), we do not necessarily receive or absorb all the nutrients listed on a food label as being contained in a given portion. This is because some nutrients are destroyed during harvesting, shipping, processing, preservation, and cooking. What we must concern ourselves with is *not* the amount of a given nutrient listed on a package, nor the amount stated as adequate for our age and weight in the RDA tables, but how much we may need as individuals, and how much reaches the cells of our body.

How to determine our individual nutrient needs is presented in detail in my previous book, *The Skeptical Nutritionist.* Here let me simply reemphasize that we may be receiving *too much* of certain nutrients (fat and protein in particular) and far, far too little of many vitamins (particularly vitamin B_6, folic acid, vitamin E, and vitamin C), and inadequate levels of essential trace minerals (particularly selenium, chromium, and zinc).

To overcome these excesses and deficiencies I suggest that we all take a "longevity formula" of vitamins and minerals, the formula varying according to our age. These supplement formulas are listed in Appendix B, "Longevity Formula."

When we become ill, of course, our nutrient needs and tolerances change. How such changes affect your child's diet is discussed in Book III, "Natural Approaches for Natural Complaints."

DIET FOR PROSPECTIVE PARENTS

NUTRITIONAL FACTORS IN STERILITY

According to the eminent specialist Dr. Samuel R. Meaker, emeritus professor of gynecology at Boston University School of Medicine, more than 12 percent of American marriages are barren, which means that at the time of his writing, nearly three million couples of reproductive age were childless owing to problems of sterility. Of course, sterility has many causes, but certainly diet and nutrition play a very important role. It is well known, for example, that malnutrition in males definitely modifies the quantity and quality of sperm production, whereas in the female the possible inactivation of estrogens by a malfunctioning liver has been shown.

Food for Fertility

DIET TO IMPROVE FERTILITY OUTLINED

We will give examples of vitamins and minerals that have effects upon both sperm production and cervical dysfunction, but first let us summarize a general diet program to ensure that your level of fertility is as high as it can be. First stated in 1928 by Dr. D. Macomber, these suggestions were later summarized by Dr. E. Cheraskin in 1968, in his book *Diet and Disease,* and they still remain a good set of guidelines. They are as follows:

(1) Be certain your protein intake is adequate.

(2) Be certain that you are consuming adequate levels of calcium, phosphorus, iodine, iron, and other trace minerals.

(3) Be certain that all known vitamins are consumed at least at the RDA level.

(4) Your water intake must be adequate.

(5) Your total calories should be at least the level of the RDA (unless you are obese or ill).

Supplements

SEMEN COUNTS IMPROVED VIA VITAMINS

There are surprisingly few studies on the effect of nutrients on human fertility, but some studies on the male have shown that sperm production is improved both qualitatively and quantitatively by supplementation with the B vitamins and vitamin E. With the use of as little as 150–200 milligrams a day of alpha-tocopherol (vitamin E), not only was the sperm count increased in men who had problems with sperm production but also there was an improvement in sperm motility and a reduction in the number of abnormal sperm. In this study, as reported by Cheraskin, it is noted that "normal semen values were achieved in 20 of the 55 males and 21 more showed improvement. Seventeen cases proved fertile. However, it should be emphasized that improved spermatogenesis is not a guarantee for conception."

The pioneering nutritionist Dr. Carlton Fredericks, who has followed thousands of pregnancies in his career, recommends the following nutritional supplements for prospective parents: a multivitamin/mineral formula, a vitamin-B-complex syrup, a concentrated form of vitamin E, wheat-germ oil, and bioflavonoids. The exact amounts needed may of course vary with individual needs, but a general insurance formula is to be found according to your age and weight in Appendix B.

RULES TO EAT BY OUTLINED

For those who plan to have children, it is important not only to include adequate levels of nutrients in the diet but also to avoid substances that may harm you or your future offspring. For this reason, you will need to consider giving up some of our civilization's most popular (and legal) drugs. Caffeine, for example, has been implicated in recent Soviet studies as a possible cause of genetic damage in infants whose *fathers* drank coffee before conception! Of course, the harmful habit of smoking that provides nicotine should also be given up, and your alcohol intake should be limited to no more than a few ounces a day, if not cut out entirely. Eliminating foods containing additives, as well as refined sugar (sucrose), from the diet will further help to lay the groundwork for the production of healthy children.

On the positive side, increase your intake of fresh fruits and vegetables, eat only whole grains (rather than refined white flour), and eat regularly. Finally, do not eat until your body has been warmed with a little brisk exercise, in order to derive the greatest benefit from your well-regulated diet.

NOURISHING THE UNBORN:
DIET IN PREGNANCY

Folk Wisdom and Folk Foolishness:
Is Intuition Enough?

WOMEN USED TO GET GOOD ADVICE FROM RELATIVES

In recent years, a great deal of attention has been paid to the diet of pregnant women. But surely, you may object, the problem can't be all that complicated. For millennia women have been bearing children without the benefit of sophisticated nutritional theories. Those women did get good advice, however. Living closer to their mothers and grandmothers, they received the benefit of life experience through a folk-nutrition network. Such folk wisdom is what this book will bring you in addition to the latest scientific information, so that you can help your child be as healthy as genetically possible. Faced with conflicting nutritional information, people often throw up their hands in despair and follow their "instincts." Although instincts might once have been nature's guides, they have been seriously modified by many subtle and some unsubtle pressures, such as advertising. To help you recognize your true instincts regarding food is one of the purposes of this section.

No area of diet is more filled with folklore than that of pregnancy. "Pica," the eating of nonfood items in response to peculiar cravings, is an example. Many women believe the developing fetus signals its nutritional needs to the mother in the form of these unusual cravings.

SOME PREGNANT WOMEN EAT CLAY, DIRT, ASHES, ETC.

In a study, anthropologists L. F. Snow and S. M. Johnson reported that expectant mothers ate clay, starch, dirt, rocks, ashes, coral, charcoal, ice cubes, baking powder, matches, and match boxes. The women claimed that their cravings represented a dietary need. One pregnant patient asserted that it was a good idea to eat healing clays because they served as "a scrub brush to the organs."

Another very unusual example of a food craving during pregnancy, reported in the same study, concerns a woman who did not smoke but who experienced a strong craving for cigarette ashes. She would carefully burn cigarettes down to the ash and then eat them with a spoon! She was quoted as saying "My first two babies were born in the eighth month, but the last two were full term. I figure the cigarette ashes made me carry the last two longer, so maybe it was a good thing to do." The woman believed her craving had identified a specific against premature birth—cigarette ashes.

SOME "HEALTH FOOD" CONCEPTS FAULTY

Unusual beliefs go beyond the ingestion of nonfood items. The same anthropologists, Snow and Johnson,* reported on a young vegetarian who stated that "you can feel what the baby needs" nutritionally. This patient described her diet during pregnancy, which changed each month according to what she interpreted to be the changing needs of the baby's development:

> She stated that the mother should also monitor her own body and, if she felt that her fingernails were becoming too thin or her teeth not strong, this could be remedied by eating increased amounts of lettuce and cabbage. She arrived at the clinic for her first prenatal visit at 31 weeks' gestation, severely anemic. She was remedying this anemia by eating avocados, which she thought especially rich in iron.

* L. F. Snow and S. M. Johnson,"Folklore, Food, Female Reproductive Cycle." *Ecology of Food and Nutrition,* Vol. 7, pp. 41–49.

Now, avocados *are* rich in iron, but unfortunately this essential nutrient is not very well absorbed from fibrous vegetable foods unless they are eaten with meat. As an example, only 2 to 5 percent of the iron found in spinach or whole wheat is absorbed from the small intestine. Beans, corn, and rice also contain iron that is poorly absorbed, but when these vegetable foods are eaten with meat, the amount of iron absorbed is doubled. For a vegetarian, then, eating avocados would be of little specific benefit in increasing the body's iron stores.

Another pregnant vegetarian in this study also thought that the diet should be altered during this time. She said that

> a pregnant woman should not eat meat, fish, or eggs, as these are "dead flesh" and "dead flesh does not regenerate." She recommended eating more fruit, vegetables, grains, sprouts, and dairy products, as these "regenerate and cleanse the body," plus a "Mama's drink" composed of vegetable juice cocktail, lemon juice and wheat germ oil, which she believed would prevent stretch marks.

DOCTRINE OF MATERNAL IMPRESSIONS

Where do these strange notions come from? Apparently, they go back to an ancient "doctrine of maternal impressions" that was based on the premise that any strong emotional feelings of the mother such as desire, sorrow, pity, anger, or fear would somehow be directly transferred to the child. More than 70 percent of the women interviewed in this Michigan study still believed in the possibility of "marking" the child through strong emotions of the mother. Some informants believed that food could mark a baby and give it red spots if the mother ate too many fruits that were red, such as strawberries or cherries. Another thought that if the mother ate a piece of chocolate, the baby would have a chocolate mark. But, by and large, most of the patients believed that a baby could be marked by an unsatisfied food craving.

While not all women have folkloric beliefs about what to eat during pregnancy, 90 percent of the prenatal patients in the above study were aware that a pregnant woman should change her diet; and of these 90 percent, 93 percent agreed that a pregnant woman should avoid "junk food such as carbonated beverages, sweets and potato chips, and eat more fresh vegetables and fruits, meat, eggs, and milk."

ETHNIC FACTOR ALSO IMPORTANT

Many factors besides nutrients must be taken into consideration. For example, ethnic and cultural differences must also be considered when evaluating the nutritional status of the mother and later of her children. For example, many Mexican Americans follow a "hot and cold theory" that leads to the avoidance and acceptance of many different foods, especially during pregnancy. Women of any ethnic group, however, must pay particular attention to their diet during pregnancy, because the mother is nurturing the child through her own body, and is subject to this additional stress.

The Scientific Approach:
The Changing Nutrient Needs of Pregnancy

OLD IDEA OF FETUS AS PARASITE

Would you believe that as recently as twenty to twenty-five years ago, medical schools taught that since the growing fetus was merely a parasite, it would get all that it needed from the mother, *regardless* of the mother's nutritional status? We now know that this is untrue; if the mother is not adequately nourished, the chances for maldevelopment of the child are great, particularly the chances for development of an underweight child, or a child with serious neurological and intellectual handicaps. There is also danger for the mother who is not properly nourished during the stressful period of pregnancy.

FIRST EIGHT WEEKS A CRITICAL TIME

It's a pity that just when a woman needs to be particularly well nourished—that is, at the time of conception—she is often in a very poor nutritional state. You see, from the time of fertilization up to the point when the placenta is largely developed, eight weeks after fertilization, the developing embryo derives all of its needs from nutrients in the mother's tissues and her secretions, and so the *prior* nutritional status of the mother is vitally important, especially during this first trimester, when most of the organs of the developing child are being laid down.

Before we go on to outline some dietary rules for pregnancy, let's take a look at how the fetus receives its nourishment.

FEEDING OCCURS ACROSS PLACENTA

Many women don't realize that there is no direct connection between the mother and fetus other than an interchange between their bloodstreams through the placenta. The blood from the mother and the fetus come close to one another in this organ, and the constituents pass through the placental membrane, from one to the other. The fetus draws in nutrients in their simplest forms and eliminates wastes at the same time.

ONLY NUTRIENTS CROSS PLACENTA, NOT MENUS

This is important to bear in mind, because no matter how fancy your meals may be, or how simple, it is only the nutrients that pass the placenta, not the menu. Certainly a carefully arranged meal may have an emotional impact on the mother that can affect pregnancy, but nutrients are nutrients, and it is these components that are of vital importance in pregnancy.

CHANGES IN MOTHER DURING FIRST THREE MONTHS OF PREGNANCY

Pregnancy has traditionally been divided into three-month periods, or trimesters. During the first trimester (months 1–3), the fetus increases so little in size that its daily need for nutrients is almost negligible; but demands are made upon the mother's body in other ways as nature adapts it for the later stages of pregnancy and eventually nursing. During this time nausea and digestive problems are frequently experienced. This is perfectly normal, and does not occur because the fetus is making demands but because of adjustments in the mother's overall physiology. Eating six small meals a day during this period rather than the three traditional full meals may prove less stressful.

It is also very wise to take a vitamin/mineral supplement during the first trimester, but it is not easy to predict categorically all of the vitamins and minerals that may be needed by all mothers. We will discuss some of the more commonly needed nutrients later in this section. One important rule is that vitamin/mineral supplements should be taken *with meals or immediately after* to avoid the nausea and vomiting that may be caused by certain formulas.

DRAMATIC SECOND-TRIMESTER CHANGES

The second trimester (months 4–6) is an extremely important phase of fetal development. During this period the mother's breasts and uterus enlarge while the amniotic fluid and placenta are being formed and the mother's blood volume increases. She also begins to put on a substantial amount of fat, which acts as a safety buffer against possible food deprivation later on in pregnancy. At about the sixth month, the developing fetus is gaining about 10 grams per day; by comparison, only 1 gram of weight per day is gained during the first trimester.

NEEDS INCREASE DURING LAST TRIMESTER

But most of the weight gain is yet to come, because fully half the total increase occurs in the eighth and ninth months, and it is during these final months of pregnancy that the diet must be nutritionally rich. It is important to continue exercise programs and to continue working and not to deny yourself the desire to eat more.While many mature women utilize approximately 2300 calories a day in the middle of their pregnancies, they use about 200–300 calories more per day during the final two and a half months, while women who work at active jobs or who have other young children in the house need even more food energy. Of course, should you be fortunate enough to be carrying twins or triplets, you will need an even greater amount of calories.

Determining Your Dietary Needs

IDEAL DIET ONLY AN ESTIMATE

Although science has found out a great deal about the nutritional requirements during pregnancy, we cannot point to an "ideal diet" that will be right for all pregnant women. Individual differences and ethnic variation would in any case invalidate such blanket prescriptions, but in addition ethical considerations preclude the human experiments that would be necessary to study this problem. It is possible to *estimate* nutritional requirements for mother and child only by studying changes in body composition and metabolism and by using other gross clinical observations.

ETHNIC DIFFERENCES REINFORCED

It should be understood immediately that ethnic differences may be so dramatic that the RDAs for the pregnant mother really only represent a norm for white women in the United States and Britain. To apply these data to other racial groups would be a medical and ethical absurdity. Nevertheless, given these limitations, we still have a fairly good idea of what a good diet is for most pregnant mothers of most ethnic groups. What we have are a set of coordinates through which we must draw a line based upon ethnic concepts of prenatal nutrition as well as more recent scientific findings.

Dietary Analysis

It is important not only that the mother receive high-quality nourishment when she knows she is pregnant but also that she be prepared nutritionally *before* pregnancy, so that she has adequate stores to take care of both herself and her child during the important early developmental stages. We know from animal experiments that several generations must receive adequate nutrition before full development can take place in the offspring, especially if the deprivations in prior generations were severe. From such evidence, it is clear that establishing proper nutrition before conception is necessary and that upon conception, the mother's nutrient needs are going to be increased to provide for the infant's proper growth and development.

HAIR AND DIETARY ANALYSIS RECOMMENDED

To be on the safe side, it is really important for a *pregnant* woman to have an assessment of her nutritional status made early on. For this purpose I recommend that a computer-generated dietary analysis, as well as a hair analysis for toxic minerals, be done by a competent nutritionist *just as soon as you know for sure that you are pregnant,* then again at four months, and then again at seven months. This method of evaluating nutritional status is available to anyone; and for preventive purposes, the mother's nutritional status should be determined, especially during the first trimester, if it has not been done before. The results of the hair analysis will show the levels of toxic metals, such as lead, mercury, and arsenic. Should any of these compounds be detected, a diet to eliminate them slowly is to be followed. By eating a high-protein diet and slow-cooked beans, we can cause chemical groups within these foods to "lock on" to the toxic metals, so that the poisons are eliminated together with the foods.

The dietary analysis is based on the mother's report of the foods she actually eats, and the computer printout will show the levels of all important nutrients in her diet. The hair analysis and dietary analysis, then, can form the basis for recommending alterations in the mother's diet and specific vitamin/mineral supplementation.

Common Deficiencies in Pregnancy and Before

VITAMINS A, B'S, C, IODINE, CALCIUM,
AND IRON IN SHORT SUPPLY

Dietary surveys of pregnant women in the United States have found, surprisingly, that all ages and economic groups show deficiencies of vitamin A, B vitamins, vitamin C, iodine, calcium, and iron. Trace minerals such as zinc and copper are also very low.

THE "PILL" INCREASES NEED FOR VITAMIN B_6

Even before pregnancy, many women may have specific deficiencies, some of them arising from their method of birth control. Women who use oral contraceptives show an increased need for vitamin B_6, and in many cases folic acid. A very common complaint among women on the pill is a serious feeling of depression. It is known that a deficiency of vitamin B_6 leads in many cases to a feeling of depression, and since the blood levels of vitamin B_6 in women on birth-control pills is lowered, large doses are sometimes necessary to bring the levels of this vitamin back up to normal. Clinical studies have shown that when large quantities of this vitamin are given, raising it back up to normal blood levels, the depression tends to lift. (50-100 mg of Vitamin B_6 as a supplement is the usual dosage.)

MANY FACTORS PRODUCE DEFICIENCIES

Women who use intrauterine contraceptive devices (IUDs) before pregnancy often experience large losses of blood on a regular basis, which tends to increase deficiencies in critical nutrients. Nutrient deficiencies may also be due to poor eating habits and limited food budgets, which encourage the consumption of cheap, refined carbohydrates such as white flour and sugar, in the form of devitalized bread, pasta, cakes, pastries, potato chips, pretzels, and other "junk food."

Consequences of Deficiencies During Pregnancy

MOTHER MAY BE HARMED

While the nutrients that are needed by the child must come from the mother's food, the developing embryo may draw them, if necessary, from the mother's tissues, even at the expense of the mother's nutritional status. A young woman who already has good food habits really has to alter her diet only slightly during pregnancy, increasing the intake of some of the foods she is already accustomed to eating and eliminating a few others. Unfortunately, many women have not developed good food habits, and so they enter pregnancy very poorly nourished, and borderline deficiences that have not previously manifested themselves often become apparent at this time.

HOW TO AVOID ANEMIA

For example, if a woman had previously had a borderline intake of iron or folacin, anemia could easily develop during pregnancy because of the extra demands of the developing fetus. In areas of the world where goiter is prevalent, latent iodine deficiency can easily be manifested during pregnancy through an enlarged thyroid gland.

TEEN PREGNANCIES A DOUBLE PROBLEM

When teenage girls become pregnant, the needs of the developing fetus and that of the developing teenager must both be considered. Unfortunately, both young mother and infant are often the losers during these pregnancies, owing to the poor eating habits of most American teenagers.

MOTHER LOSES TEETH

An extreme example of the consequences of a borderline deficiency occurred in one of my clients during an earlier pregnancy. Long before I came to know this woman, she had borne a child at great expense to her own health. She lost sixteen of her teeth during pregnancy, and not one physician or even her dentist thought it was related to her pregnancy! When she came to see me years later, we pieced the story together as follows. This woman had always abhorred dairy products, exhibiting the classic symptoms of lactase insufficiency; that is, she did not have the enzyme lactase required to digest lactose or milk sugar; therefore, she was unable to digest significant quantities of milk or dairy products, an extremely important source of calcium. When the developing fetus drew on the mother's calcium stores, which were already insufficient, she lost her teeth. As a postscript, the infant was born and lost all her teeth. Had the obstetrician or pediatrician or dentist attending this woman and her baby been aware of nutritional factors, they would have recognized the symptoms of lactase insufficiency and arranged for her to eat large quantities of fermented dairy products, which do not require that lactase be digested. Foods such as yogurt would have been capable of reversing this serious problem. Calcium supplementation should also have been recommended, in the form of calcium-magnesium tablets and/or dolomite powder or pills.

SOME SPONTANEOUS ABORTION, STILLBIRTH PREVENTABLE

Nutritional deficiencies can also lead to complications for the mother during and before birth, and to premature birth, spontaneous abortion, stillbirth, or neonatal death of the infant. In an excellent survey of this subject in his book *Diet and Disease,* Dr. E. Cheraskin observes that 10 percent of deaths in the United States "occur during or immediately after gestation." He estimates that half of these losses of life are preventable and considers dietary deficiencies to be leading contributing factors. Studies have shown that among women with poor diets, an increase in the intake of protein, B vitamins, vitamin C, bioflavonoids, iodine, and vitamin E helps to reduce obstetrical complications.

Cheraskin reports that an interesting and apparently paradoxical effect has been observed among some populations during wartime, when normal food supplies were reduced. In spite of decreased food supplies, there was a lower incidence of toxemia among pregnant women during these wartime periods. It has been suggested that the pregnant women received extra rations of important nutrients such as milk and vitamin supplements, or possibly that their diets under these conditions were closer to those of "primitive" peoples, containing fewer refined foods, less animal fat and protein, more fruit and vegetables. Such a diet, low in fat and often low in calories, is often distinctly richer in vitamin and mineral content.

INDIAN DIET HEALTHFUL

Indeed, it appears that for all our sophisticated nutritional knowledge, isolated, primitive peoples often enjoy superior health, and this may become particularly apparent during pregnancy and birth. Cheraskin reports that a study of the Indians of British Columbia during the years 1925–1929 revealed an incidence of stillbirth of 1.26 percent, as compared to 2.73 percent for the white population of British Columbia and 2.09 percent for all of Canada during the same period! Yet the Indian mothers generally delivered their babies without the benefit of medical assistance and subsisted on diets consisting primarily of salmon, salmon eggs, and seaweed (a rich source of iodine). Clearly we do not yet have all the answers in the important area of prenatal nutrition.

A Dietary Plan for Pregnancy

Having looked at the background of nutritional requirements during pregnancy, we can now outline a diet. The best course to follow is for the mother to receive all of her recommended dietary allowances plus an allowance for pregnancy (see Appendix A for amounts).

This additional allowance will vary, but in general an increase between 15 and 30 percent of all nutrients is necessary, with particular emphasis on protein, calories, vitamins, and minerals.

"FOOD FASCISM" DISAVOWED

Not believing in that form of "food fascism" that dictates specific meal plans *ad infinitum*, I have found it best to suggest groups of foods and to leave the specific amounts and proportions to the person's own choosing. This works best because people who are not forced to follow a diet will enjoy their food more and tend to eat more nutritiously. But please bear in mind that these nutrient requirements are extremely important. Any harm done owing to dietary deficits during the period of brain development, which usually extends from about the third month of pregnancy through at least the second or third year of life, is irreparable! This means that the diet must be nutritionally adequate for the mother during pregnancy, during nursing, and for the infant during the early years of life.

OMNIVOROUS DIET RECOMMENDED

The rules for eating during pregnancy are really the rules for eating on a daily basis. I always recommend an omnivorous diet that emphasizes fruits, vegetables, nuts, legumes, whole grains, cheese, milk, eggs, occasionally meat, poultry without skin, and fish. Sugary desserts should be avoided because they are poor in nutrition and add weight at the same time. If you get a craving for sweets, chop up a fruit salad, put some raw honey on it, and sprinkle a little wheat germ on top. It is one of the finest desserts available. Or try some of the recipes for "sweet things" in Book IV, "Recipes for Resisters."
The "Diet for Prospective Parents" section, pp.5-7,

outlines a sensible program for good nutrition. Here are the nutrients you will require during pregnancy:

Dairy. Approximately one quart of yogurt or low-fat milk per day. You may substitute at the rate of 1½ oz. of cheddar cheese per glass of milk. Remember also that cheese contains whey, a very important dietary component. ("He who fifes and eats his whey will live to fife another day.") Cheese is also a good calcium source for people who are allergic to dairy products owing to a lactase deficiency; you'll know you're allergic if you experience stool softening or excessive intestinal gas when you drink milk. Cheese and yogurt have had the lactose they contain broken down during fermentation by microorganisms, and are good alternative calcium sources, if you are lactase-deficient.

There are alternatives to dairy products for calcium. These include dark, leafy green vegetables (particularly broccoli and cauliflower); fish bones, which are eaten when you eat salmon, sardines, smelt, or other dried fish; sesame seeds, a common ingredient of Near Eastern cookery; and tahini (a very tasty sesame-seed paste). But bear in mind that the plant sources of calcium lack vitamin B_{12}, which must be added from other sources.

Fleshy Foods. For nonvegetarians about 8 oz. (cooked weight) of meat, fish, or poultry should be eaten on a daily basis. Once a week some liver or other organ meat is recommended. Those who do not eat meat may substitute beans, peas, lentils, eggs, and cheese.

Fruits and Vegetables. You will need approximately four bountiful portions daily, particularly dark, leafy green vegetables. Be certain that one of these portions contains a vitamin-C-rich food, such as orange, lemon, lime, grapefruit, papaya, melon, tomato, or cabbage. Many dishes can be supplemented with green or red peppers, which are highly concentrated sources of vitamin C.

Cereals and Breads. Eat about four slices of true whole-grain bread a day; or if you do not care to eat bread, substitute for each slice of bread about ½ to ⅔ cup of cooked whole-wheat cereal, baked potatoes, or mashed potatoes. If you use pasta, please make certain it is whole-wheat pasta.

Fats and Oils. I highly recommend that butter and margarine be avoided—butter because of the coloring that is frequently added; margarine because of the hydrogenated oil and synthetic flavorings and colorings. It is much better to use sunflower-seed oil, safflower oil, or corn oil. Olive oil can be used occasionally for taste. Of course, this category can be almost entirely eliminated if you use milk and dairy products; in that case you will need only 1 tablespoonful of one of these linoleic-acid-rich vegetable oils.

Vitamin and Mineral Supplements

HAIR AND DIET ANALYSIS A GUIDE TO SUPPLEMENTATION

The hair analysis, in conjunction with a computer-generated dietary analysis, should give the mother-to-be and her attending obstetrician an opportunity to decide which if any supplements are required during pregnancy, especially during the first trimester. If these tests reveal all nutrient levels to be adequate, you should still consider the following supplementation, if you are not hypersensitive to any of these nutrients:

Iron: 15–60 mg. (milligrams) daily; *calcium:* 2 grams of a nonphosphate calcium salt daily*; *folic acid:* 800 mcg. (micrograms) a day; *zinc:* 15–20 mg. daily. *Iodine:* use iodized salt, or take a prenatal multivitamin/mineral formula that contains some iodine.

---

*This calcium supplementation is recommended only for those women who do not eat milk, cheese, or other dairy products, or who are lactose-intolerant and avoid dairy products entirely.

VEGETARIAN WOMEN MUST HAVE A B₁₂ SUPPLEMENT

Vegetarian women, especially strict vegetarians who eat no milk, eggs, fish, or poultry, are absolutely going to need a vitamin-B_{12} supplement to prevent damage to their infants' central nervous systems.

ALL IRON-RICH FOODS NOT ABSORBABLE

If you plan to breast-feed your baby, remember that human milk is low in iron and copper, and so your developing baby must be supplied with these minerals during your pregnancy in order for his liver to have a sufficient reserve to last through the early months of nursing. Unless the pregnancy diet is iron- and copper-rich, the baby and mother will become anemic. Traditional obstetricians generally prescribe approximately 15 mg. of iron per day for the pregnant mother. However, some women are allergic to iron and are unable to take supplements. In these cases it is always advisable that foods rich in absorbable iron be emphasized in the diet. Good sources of absorbable iron include broiled lamb liver, beef liver, chicken, molasses, soybeans, apricots, prunes, figs, and raisins.

CALCIUM-RICH FOODS

Calcium, of course, is one of the most important foods for pregnant and nursing mothers, and milk and other dairy sources as well as vegetable sources of calcium must be consumed in large quantities to avoid mineral depletion and possible tooth loss. If the mother is allergic to milk and dairy products, or for any other reason does not use them, supplementation is absolutely mandatory in the form of dolomite powder or calcium/magnesium tablets. *Excellent* sources of calcium are soft fish bones (in salmon, sardines, herring); dark, leafy green vegetables; milk; and hard cheeses. *Good* sources include dried figs, dried legumes, broccoli, baked beans, and softer cheeses.

Folic acid is another nutritional need in pregnancy, and a supplementary 0.3–0.4 mg. is generally prescribed. However, this is a rather low quantity, and foods rich in folic acid should also be emphasized during pregnancy. The following table lists some good sources of folic acid.

TABLE 1
Some Foods Rich in Folic Acid*

Food (about 100 grams)	Approximate Cooking Portion	Total Folacin (micrograms)
Garbanzo beans	1 cup	398
Soybeans, dry	1 cup	359
Yeast, brewer's	1 tbsp.	313
Yeast, baker's dry	1 pkg.	286
Spinach, cooked	1 cup	164
Peanuts, roasted	1 cup	153
Almonds	1 cup	136
Orange juice	1 cup	136
Wheat germ, toasted	1 oz.	118
Ground beef, cooked (for comparison)	3 oz.	3

*After Briggs & Calloway (1979).

MEAT, FRUIT, POOR SOURCES OF FOLIC ACID

The foods itemized above are just a sample. Other good sources of folacin (folic acid) are green vegetables (broccoli, lettuce, cabbage, etc.), nuts, whole oranges, and whole grains. *Poor* sources include eggs (22 micrograms per 100 grams), meats, most fruits, potatoes, dried milk, desserts, and white flour.

Leafy greens, while good sources of folacin, can lose up to 70 percent of this vitamin if stored at room temperature for only three days. Similarly, cooking destroys up to 65 percent of folic acid present in foods. So you must consume fresh, uncooked foods as much as possible to make sure you are getting the RDA of 800 micrograms daily needed during pregnancy.

PROTEIN SUPPLEMENTS NOT ADVISED

Of course, adequate protein intake is extremely important during pregnancy. A study in the United States has shown that mothers who were on a low protein intake experienced an increased incidence of spontaneous abortion, while those mothers who had up to about 90 grams per day of positive protein intake delivered infants of good weight, size, and well-being. A well-balanced diet must contain *adequate* levels of protein. It is absurd to take protein supplements while pregnant, because protein added to a diet cannot be utilized properly if the overall calories are restricted.

Nutritional Solutions to Problems of Pregnancy

MORNING SICKNESS TREATED WITH VITAMIN B₆

The best cure is prevention, and nausea during pregnancy is best prevented by following the "Diet for Prospective Parents" outlined earlier and including supplements. If morning sickness or pregnancy nausea does crop up, you can reduce or completely control the symptoms by taking about 30 mg. of vitamin B₆ in addition to vitamin-B-complex supplement. If digestive disturbances occur, especially during the last stages of pregnancy, and interfere with your ability to eat enough food to meet your daily requirements, try changing to six small meals a day and taking more liquid foods rich in nutrients, such as malteds made with a rich source of malt; fruit drinks with added yeast and/or wheat germ; milk drinks, perhaps with added egg; and other concentrated foods.

VITAMIN C CAN REDUCE RISK OF VARICOSE VEINS

Varicose veins is another common problem that may result from the extra weight you are carrying, and also because the fetus draws a large amount of vitamin C from your own supply. To offset this extra demand and reduce the risk of developing bulging, unsightly veins, increase your intake of vitamin C, vitamin E, the B complex, and fiber. All of these nutrients, except the fiber, will be present in a good quality vitamin/mineral prenatal formula. The relationship between varicose veins and these nutritional factors is reported by Dr. Carlton Fredericks in *Food Facts and Fallacies,* and is based on his observation of thousands of pregnancies. For the skeptical obstetrician, further information on this problem can be found in "Report on the Relation of Vitamin C Deficiency to Varicose Veins," *Western Journal of Surgery, Obstetrics, and Gynecology,* Vol. 50, 1942.

If you experience a swelling of the ankles or any other tissue, you should discuss with your obstetrician an increase in the amount of protein foods you should eat, adding up to 5 additional ounces a day of such foods as fish, poultry, meat, eggs, and dairy.

RIBOFLAVIN AND HEARTBURN

Heartburn is another common complaint, usually in the fifth month. This has traditionally been relieved by injections of vitamin B_2, or riboflavin. The reason why women need more of this nutrient is that at this time the baby draws more heavily from the mother's supplies, just when the mother herself has increased needs for riboflavin.

What to Avoid

TOBACCO, ADDITIVES, DRUGS, ALCOHOL, ARE POISONS

Nearly as important as the foods you eat are the potentially dangerous substances you should avoid during pregnancy. Restricting or eliminating your alcohol intake is one of the important steps you must take to ensure optimal health for your baby. Women who drink alcohol heavily tend to deliver babies with smaller than normal heads, babies of subnormal mentality, babies with abnormal facial features, and babies who experience deficient growth.

Smoking is an equally harmful habit. Those who smoke generally deliver babies of lower birth weight than do nonsmokers. The white-blood-cell counts are elevated in smokers even when they are not suffering from infection, and their blood clots much more quickly than that of nonsmokers. Protein, which is so important to the developing embryo and to the health of the mother, is also affected by smoking; it has been known for over forty years that smoking impairs protein metabolism while increasing the amount of cholesterol in the blood. The loss of bone mineral often experienced by smokers may possibly be related to the loss of vitamin C caused by smoking, and toxic trace metals that are found in smoke can accumulate in the body and adversely affect the developing fetus. Present in tobacco leaves are arsenic, lead, cadmium, and radioactive polonium. These are all good reasons for avoiding the use of tobacco, especially while pregnant. Moreover, tobacco is known to interact with a number of drugs, speeding up the process by which the body eliminates them. Of course, you should not be taking any drugs during pregnancy without good medical reason, but if you are a smoker and are taking pentazocine, imipramine, theophylline, glutethimide, or furosemide, your doctor may need to adjust your dosage. The obvious message is to quit smoking, for your baby's sake and for your own!

To repeat, avoid *all* medications during pregnancy, even aspirin, unless specifically ordered by your physician. Avoid exposure to environmental contaminants, including chemicals and radiation (including X ray). Read food labels carefully and avoid any foods that contain chemical additives or preservatives.

About Salt Intake and Weight Gain

Many women worry about water retention and weight gain during pregnancy.

BIRTH DEFECTS NOT CAUSED BY SALT

We know of no reason to restrict salt intake. Pregnant women will frequently experience some retention of salt and water because of the high levels of hormones manufactured during pregnancy that influence the salt and water content of the body. This in no way signifies any danger to the mother. In fact, if anything, proper nutrition including adequate salt intake will probably decrease the chances of developing complications, including eclampsia, rather than have any adverse effect.

REASONABLE WEIGHT GAIN DEFINED

Nor is there any reason for excessive concern about weight gain during pregnancy. Remember this: a normal weight gain during pregnancy ranges between 24 and 28 pounds, and complications occur more frequently among women who are greatly overweight or seriously underweight *at the time of conception,* and among those who deviate *greatly* from the normal rate of gain. Of course, women who are particularly thin will have to gain more than the average amount of weight during pregnancy. A standard rule of thumb is that weight gain be spaced out at about 4 pounds during the first trimester, 10 pounds during the second trimester, and 10 pounds during the third trimester; but of course norms are just that, and variations should and do occur.

A Positive Approach to Proper Nutrition

A cardinal rule to remember is that you can't ensure proper nutrition simply by eliminating dangerous chemicals from your diet while subsisting on a meager intake or a diet of junk foods. It will not work. You must eat a well-balanced diet if you want to have a well-balanced baby. For a more complete description of foods to eat and foods to avoid, Book II, "The Diet of Older Children," describes the dangers inherent in everyday foods, tells how to avoid them, and what foods are advisable— for adults as well as for children.

HOW TO USE OUR RECIPES

In Book IV, "Recipes for Resisters," you will find meals and dishes intended for youngsters resistant to most "healthy" foods. It contains a very wide selection of meals that are excellent to incorporate into your diet at the time of pregnancy. Everything from types of breads, sample breakfasts, main dishes, gravies and sauces, dressings and spreads, vegetables, soups, sweets, to some helpful tips for healthful food preparation is fully outlined for your use. Bear in mind that these recipes, which come from the Weimar Institute, in California, are all made without the use of fats or oils, sugar, dairy products, or meats. These dietary items occur too frequently in the American diet to begin with; however, since pregnancy increases the demands for calcium and for some oils that contain linoleic acid, you must be willing to use foods that contain these nutrients. So, should you *not* be a vegetarian, you can use our menus to *supplement* your diet, at the same time eliminating all sugar and foods containing sugar.

NURSING

Human Milk—The Perfect Infant Food

NATURAL APPROACH TO BIRTH AND FEEDING PREFERRED

By now everyone knows that breast milk is the perfect infant food. After several decades of technological flirtation and an attempt to persuade us that formula or cow's milk is better, we now see the pendulum swinging back to a more natural approach to infant nutrition. People are once again recognizing the truth in the maxim "You can't improve on nature." As more women are choosing to avoid anesthesia, electing instead various natural childbirth approaches such as the Leboyer method, so also they are returning to breast-feeding. Even though attempts are constantly being made to refine various formulas and to make them mimic human milk more closely, none of them has yet equaled it, for human milk contains many protective factors and uniquely adapted nutrient balances that cannot be supplied by any formula.

It is well known that each species has unique requirements, and each mammalian species has evolved a milk finely tuned to the needs of its newborn. The ratios of the various nutrients in the composition of the milk of any species are related to the pace at which the newborn is expected to grow.

COW'S MILK EVOLVED FOR RAPID WEIGHT GAIN

When we compare cow's milk with human milk, we see that they meet quite different needs. Cow's milk has been developed over millions of years for the growing calf, which is supposed to double its birth weight in a third of the time that it takes for a human infant to do so; and so cow's milk is more highly concentrated in protein and other building materials. Looking at Table 2, we see that cow's milk contains about three times as much protein as human milk, and is also much more highly concentrated in calcium and phosphorus. Looking more carefully, we notice that the calcium-phosphorus ratio in human milk is approximately 3:1, while in cow's milk it is only 1.5:1. Again, the relative growth rates between baby calves and baby humans explain these differences. Look at the higher amount of niacin in human milk as compared to cow's milk, and the much higher value for vitamin C; human milk contains about four times as much vitamin C as cow's milk. Human milk is quite a bit richer in fat and sugar (lactose) than cow's milk; and to return to the proteins again, the table shows that of the total protein, cow's milk has twice the casein found in human milk, while human milk contains three times the whey proteins of cow's milk.

FAT AND SUGAR IN HUMAN MILK CRITICAL

These differences, as we have said, reflect the different rates of growth. Baby humans have a much higher growth rate of their central nervous system during the first year of life, and a relatively low rate of muscle growth. The high fat and sugar content are there to supply the requirements of newborn and very young infants, and the relatively lower protein content is sufficient for the slower rate of muscular growth in human infants, who are also slower to attain independence than are calves. (In fact, during gestation and early infancy the brain utilizes oxygen and nitrogen at a rate twice that of adults—which makes nutrition during this period of key importance for the future of the baby's intelligence and behavior.)

TABLE 2
Content of Mature Human Milk and Cow's Milk*

Composition	Human Milk	Cow's Milk
Water/100 ml	87.1	87.3
Energy: kcal[†]/100 ml	75	69
Total solids, g/100 ml	12.9	12.7
Protein	1.1	3.3
Fat	4.5	3.7
Lactose	6.8	4.8
Ash	0.21	0.72
Proteins: % of total protein		
Casein	40	82
Whey proteins	60	18
Ash, major components/l		
Calcium (mg)	340	1250
Phosphorus (mg)	140	960
Vitamins/l		
Vitamin A (IU)	1898	1025
Thiamin	160	440
Riboflavin	360	1750
Niacin	1470	940
Vitamin C (mg)	43	11
Sodium		high

*From *Nutrition and Cancer*, Vol. 1, No. 1.
†kcal is generally referred to as "calories."

It is not generally known that the human fetus and the premature newborn infant lack the enzyme cystathionase in their liver, and so they cannot utilize the amino acid methionine. Thus the human fetus and premature baby have to rely upon cystine as the essential sulfur-containing amino acid. Through a wise series of evolutionary adaptations, human milk has the lowest methionine-to-cystine ratio among all sources of animal protein. While meat, cow's milk, and other animal proteins have a methionine-to-cystine ratio ranging from 2:1 to 5:1, the ratio in human milk is nearly 1:1. Human milk is also richer in linoleic acid than is cow's milk. The absorption of this and other fatty acids supplies energy for the baby and also supports the laying down of nerves—another nutritionally specific advantage of human milk.

Human milk has the precise balance of nucleotides that enhances nitrogen uptake when protein intake is low and gives the human infant a higher rate of efficiency in utilizing the relatively low-protein milk. When we compare breast-fed and bottle-fed newborn infants, we see evidence that breast-fed infants utilize iron more efficiently. Even though breast-fed infants take in less iron during the first nine months of life than do formula-fed infants, both have similar hemoglobin values, serum-iron levels, and transferrin saturation.

COLOSTRUM CONTAINS IMMUNE SUBSTANCES

Immediately after delivery the infant should be given the breast as early as possible, for it is very critical that your child receive the colostrum, that first flow of yellowish milk that contains many of the immune substances. Extensive studies of infants of similar socioeconomic backgrounds during the first nine months of life support the conclusion that antibodies are transmitted by human milk and that the incidence of respiratory and gastrointestinal infection is much lower in breast-fed infants.

Another desirable characteristic of human milk is that it favors the development of beneficial strains of bacteria. Human milk, once it is hydrolyzed in the stomach, frees compounds that speed up the growth of *Lactobacillus bifidus.* This well-known intestinal bacterium greatly enhances the availability of vitamins and amino acids because it has metabolic processes that humans lack.

Later on in life, when the infant is given cow's milk, or in fact when anyone uses cow's milk, including the nursing mother and older children, it is wise to look for milk that contains *Lactobacillus*. In addition to enhancing the utilization of vitamins and amino acids, this bacterium helps to protect the wall of the intestine, which, it is thought, reduces tendencies toward disease.

The Importance of Breast-Feeding

SOCIAL PRESSURES AGAINST NURSING

We often hear the argument that it's difficult to nurse babies in our society, particularly for the working mother. Many women are "ashamed" to expose their breasts in public places in order to nurse. In fact, we might say that the obstacles to nursing really are almost insurmountable in our society as it is presently constructed, unless the mother desires to stay out of the workplace to care for her child. These obstacles can be removed only after women demand their right to nurse freely wherever and whenever their infant desires to eat during the initial phases of growth.

THE VALUE OF HUMAN CONTACT

By saying that human milk is the perfect food, we don't mean to imply that a mother who cannot breast-feed her infant should feel guilty or fearful that she may potentially damage her infant. Many children have developed well and normally on formula diets, but the closeness established between the mother and child during the course of nursing creates an ideal situation for the total development of the child. The mother who cannot nurse her child really must go out of her way to provide the touching, the warmth and caring, that are otherwise absent in bottle-feeding.

Problems with Formulas

SOY-MILK FORMULAS NOT PERFECT

The purpose of this book is to describe the art of feeding children naturally, leaving the "science" of feeding children to formula manufacturers. But we must recognize some important points about certain of these formulas. Soy-protein infant formulas have recently entered the marketplace in great number, as a result of concern over possible allergic problems related to cow's-milk proteins, but two major problems with soy milk have recently become public knowledge. One manufacturer with good intentions reduced the sodium content in the formula, but also unintentionally eliminated all the chloride as well. An epidemic of metabolic alkalosis in infants resulted because the formula was nutritionally deficient, and frequently no other foods were given to supplement it. Even a little fruit juice or a small meat-feeding or one banana a day would have made up for this chloride deficiency. A second indication that soy formulas are inadequate is that rickets has been observed in infants with very low birth weights who are fed exclusively on soy "milk." Soybean formulas may work well with term infants when supplemented with other foods, but are definitely to be avoided with low-birth-weight premature babies. Rickets is probably the result of an inadequate phosphorus content in addition to a vitamin-D deficiency and low calcium.

SCURVY IN CHILDREN FED ONLY ON COW'S MILK

Another danger threatens infants who are not breast-fed when mothers try to bypass formulas altogether and give unsupplemented cow's milk for the first six to twelve months: scurvy often results.

How can you tell if your baby has scurvy? The first signs of this vitamin-C deficiency are irritability, weight loss, and a lack of desire to eat. Pain on movement and a certain tenderness of the extremities are almost always present. Hemorrhages in the gums, mucous membranes, skin, and under the long bones often occur. An X ray of the long bones, though a good diagnostic aid in such cases, is not recommended, because of possible harmful effects of radiation. If these symptoms are noted, discuss them with your pediatrician, and with proper treatment an improved appetite and a better disposition can be attained within one or two days. The usual dose of vitamin C is 100 mg. a day until improvement occurs, and then 50 mg. a day until all signs disappear. (The RDA for infants is 35 mg. of vitamin C per day.)

When Not to Breast-Feed

NURSING SOMETIMES NOT ADVISABLE

Mothers who are taking medication may be advised not to breast-feed, while others who are in a somewhat weakened condition may not produce enough milk for their babies. Another rare contraindication to the use of breast milk is found when a mother develops hyperbilirubinemia. This disorder is caused by the presence of a steroid compound called pregnane-3 (alpha), 20 (beta)-diol, which inhibits the activity of an important liver enzyme in the newborn baby. Finally, in certain infant illness breast-feeding should be discontinued at least temporarily. This is more fully discussed in Book III, "Natural Approaches for Natural Complaints."

Caring for Your Breasts and Nipples

"VIRGIN" BREAST NOT PREPARED FOR NURSING

Many young mothers mistakenly believe that nature provides all that is necessary, both in birth and in feeding of the newborn. But it is a fact that many women under the age of twenty-five have "virgin" breasts, and their nipples are not sufficiently drawn out to allow a child to suckle from them, particularly during the first days of life when the baby's powers of suction are not yet strongly developed. As a result, mothers may experience much trouble during this early period of lactation. One of the ways to overcome this is by using artificial breast pumps. In earlier times women often let an older child temporarily suck on their breasts. In these cases the nipple is very likely to become fissured, and suckling can become a painful process that the mother comes to dread.

To avoid such problems, the nipples should be prepared ahead of time for their function. One effective method is to sponge the nipples carefully every night and every morning with an astringent lotion to overcome the delicacy of the skin (this should be initiated about two months prior to delivery). Another is to bring the nipples out through the use of breast shields. These are available commercially, and are often used with great advantage both prior to and during pregnancy, because they tend to lengthen the nipple and make it more easily grasped by the suckling infant. This also protects the sore nipple against rubbing or any external injury.

REMEDY FOR SORE NIPPLES

Should sore nipples develop during nursing, there are some soothing applications that can be used without harm to mother or infant. In mild cases, gum, honey, or some kind of balsam can be applied with a camel's-hair brush just after the child has been suckled. Such sores can also be healed with melted mutton fat (believe it or not!), which is applied warm in the same manner and then allowed to cool.

Diet for Nursing Mothers

SIMPLE FOODS EMPHASIZED

Recognizing the importance of providing your baby with breast milk as the ideal food, you may want to know how to eat to produce the best quality milk for your baby. The emphasis is on simplicity but generosity, including plenty of fluids. Three regular meals are advisable, consisting of milk and dairy products or calcium substitutes as discussed previously, eggs, fruits, vegetables, and much fruit and vegetable juice and filtered water or pure spring water. Whole-grain cereals and soups are highly recommended, as are the bean and lentil dishes and other recipes found in Book IV. It is important that a nursing mother avoid sour fruits, bitter salad herbs, pastry, and almost all desserts, as well as potentially allergenic foods. If meat is eaten, it should be limited to but once a day. Tea or coffee should be drastically restricted or eliminated, and only small amounts of wine or beer are recommended.

Under no circumstances should hard liquor or liqueurs be used. Remember that nutrients are not the only substances that are passed on to the baby through the milk, and so any foods containing additives, preservatives, or chemicals of any kind should be strictly avoided. This includes all artificially sweetened foods and artificial sweeteners. Even aspirin, laxatives, and sedatives pass into milk, and should be restricted unless absolutely required by a physician's orders.

OTHER FACTORS IN MOTHER'S LIFE

Besides diet, there are other things that are also important in the life of a nursing mother. During this wondrous time, you should attempt to spend some time out of doors every day, and your life, if possible, should be simple and natural. Emphasis should be placed on regular bowel movements, and rest at night should be disturbed by others as little as possible. Certainly an early bedtime is to be recommended, and by all means do take a one-hour nap in the middle of the day. You see, the emotional condition of the mother also affects the quality of the milk. Worry, anxiety, fatigue, loss of sleep, household cares, and social dissipation have a great deal to do with the failure of a nursing mother. Violent emotions, such as excitement, grief, fright, or passion, can cause milk to disagree with the child. In fact, emotional disturbances can induce an illness in the mother, and at other times can even bring about a sudden and complete disappearance of the milk supply.

Some Frequently Asked Questions About Nursing

How do we know if a nursing infant is well fed?
Your instincts will tell you. Your child will sleep two or three hours after nursing, or, if awake, is fairly quiet, good-natured, and seems to be comfortable. Color is good. Bowel movements are normal. Weight gain is slow but steady.

How do we know if a nursing child is not being properly nourished?
Such a child will not gain and may even lose some weight. Its energy level will be low, it will be fretful and irritable and will not sleep well. The child will be anemic and pale-looking. Tissues will be soft and flabby. If the milk is poor in quality or quantity, the baby will nurse for a very long time at the breast, sometimes up to three quarters of an hour, before stopping. At other times it may take the breast only for a moment and then turn away.

What should be done in such cases?
This depends on how severe the symptoms are and how long they have been present. If the child has not

gained weight for a couple of weeks or is losing weight, we suggest immediate weaning. In any case, supplementary foods in addition to the breast milk should be given at once. You can begin by alternating nursing with bottle-feeding and slowly increase the amount of bottle-feedings, or you can continue to nurse as before and give a small bottle-feeding as soon as the child is taken from the breast. Remember, though, that the quantity of the breast milk will probably be further reduced if you lessen the number of times you nurse, while more frequent nursings tend to increase the milk flow.

How do we know if the mother's milk disagrees with the child?
The symptoms are really easy to recognize. No sensitive mother can overlook a child who is sleeping little and is restless, or cries a great deal, or is constantly belching or passing gas from the bowels, or is crying from colicky pain. Surely we could not overlook vomiting or constipation or bowel movements that are frequent, loose, green, filled with mucus, and passed with much gas.

How can we correct such a situation?
If these symptoms have gone on for a couple of weeks and the child has not gained weight, and it's unlikely that the situation will be improved, breast-feeding should be stopped at once and the pediatrician consulted for a good formula. If there is a little bit of weight gain, you can keep trying for a little longer, and you can try to improve your milk flow through rest, fresh air, adjustment of diet, and the use of recipes and herbs as described on page 44. But remember, this type of trouble usually lies with the milk and not with the child.

Is there any objection to partly nursing and partly bottle-feeding a baby?
None whatever. In fact, after the first few months it may be better to bottle-feed the baby during the night in

order not to disturb the mother's sleep. But even if you have only enough milk for two or three nursings a day, these should be continued so long as the baby favors the breast milk, because even a small amount of good human milk greatly improves your child's nutrition, for the reasons discussed earlier.

Does menstruation affect the milk?

In most cases the quantity of milk is reduced, and so the infant is often not satisfied and doesn't gain as much weight. In other cases milk quality is also affected, which may cause disturbances in digestion such as restlessness, colic, and bowel changes. A few nursing infants experience acute indigestion when the mother is menstruating.

Is the return of menstruation a good reason to stop nursing?

Not always, because as a rule both functions do not go on at the same time. If your child is gaining weight regularly between the periods, nursing can be continued almost indefinitely, but it may be advisable to feed your infant with other foods in whole or in part during the first day or two of the menses.

How should the mother's diet be changed if a nursing infant habitually vomits?

If this occurs almost immediately after nursing, it usually indicates that your infant has eaten too much, and the next time you should shorten the stay at the breast, or you can give only one breast instead of two, or you can interrupt feeding by occasional rests so that the milk is not consumed too greedily. If, on the other hand, the vomiting occurs some time considerably after nursing and continues, it's a sign of indigestion, possibly because the milk is too rich in fat. In this case you should lengthen the intervals between nursings to three or even four hours, and you may consider diluting your breast milk by giving one or two tablespoons of plain boiled water, lime water, or other such water five or ten minutes prior to nursing. By shortening the nursing period you will avoid the high fat content of the later milk. Another way to reduce the fat content of the milk is to eat much less fatty foods, completely avoiding rich meats and switching more to the grains, lentils, and other such foods found in the menus in Book IV. If your baby continues to lose weight from repeated vomiting, it is usually advisable to begin weaning.

How can we treat the infant with habitual colic?

It is important in this case for the mother to try to eliminate if possible the causes of worry in her life. She should spend more time out of doors in peaceful surroundings, and eat less meat. Remember this: if you can eliminate the constipation that often accompanies colic, the colic will usually also disappear. Good herbal teas for colic are the anise, fennel, or chamomile teas described in Book III under "Colic."

How can we control constipation in a nursing infant?

By increasing the amount of milk and fresh vegetables that a mother eats, you can sometimes eliminate this situation. But remember, a mother's bowel movements should be regular and her digestion particularly attended to.

What about a nursing infant who refuses to take the breast?

This can be a serious sign. If it occurs suddenly in a child who has previously been a happy nurser, it is usually a sign of acute illness, and it is advised that you see a pediatrician at once. But if a child by degrees takes less and less of the breast until finally it won't nurse at all, you can be certain, if the child otherwise looks healthy, that there is little or no milk in the breasts. Some herbal and dietary approaches for improving milk output will now be described.

How to Increase the Quantity and Quality of Milk Through Diet and Herbal Recipes

One of the most distressing things that can happen during nursing is for the milk to be inadequate, too thin, or to dry up entirely. Let us emphasize that defective lactation in most cases is definitely curable, and with proper treatment the mother can handle the problem, not only without stressing herself but with great advantage to her baby.

TOTAL VEGETARIAN DIET CAN PRODUCE "THIN" MILK

Diet. The first and best course of treatment for defective lactation is to adjust the diet. One of the best ways to increase the flow of milk in all animals is to give them an abundant amount of food, and this is also one of the best ways to increase the milk flow in female humans. While the quantity of food eaten is often carefully monitored by pediatricians, strict attention must be paid to its quality as well. Not only is it necessary to produce a sufficient amount of milk; the milk must also be rich in nutrients. In this respect the consumption of a diet that is exclusively composed of vegetables may be insufficient. A totally vegetarian diet tends to make the milk thin. Only when leguminous plants or the higher cereals or meats and fleshy foods are eaten—that is, when a good quantity of foods containing nitrogen is taken—does both the quantity and the quality of the milk improve.

CERTAIN FOODS PROMOTE BREAST MILK

Traditional recipes and foods. There are many recipes for improving milk supply. One of the most frequently mentioned is whiting soup, but other fish that are rich in phosphorus are beneficial. Crab is also a very popular home remedy for this problem, but you must be very cautious, especially in the first months of nursing, because foods such as crabs and oysters when passed through the milk, sometimes disagree with the infant and may produce negative results. When no adverse effects are observed, these seafoods can be eaten and can benefit both mother and child.

We quote here an early recipe from France for improving the quality and quantity of milk:

> Combine three pounds of conger eel and two calves' feet with two quarts of water. Boil gently until the first is reduced to rags, then strain and add sweet herbs and asparagus or peas, a pint of milk, a piece of butter the size of a walnut, with a little flour to thicken. When used as a galactagogue [milk stimulator], use fennel in lieu of sweet herbs and haricot beans in lieu of the asparagus.

Other kinds of solid food and fleshy products have been recommended through the ages, and since one of the objects of this book is to pass on some folk wisdom regarding diet in pregnancy and in nursing and the art of feeding children, we include them here.

Lentil, pea, and bean soups have a marked effect on improving both the flow and the richness of milk. Lentils and beans are preferable to peas because the peas sometimes produce gas, either in the mother or the child. Both turnips and potatoes have been known to improve the mother's milk supply, and mushrooms, which are rich in nitrogen, also increase the quantity of milk.

BEER AS A MILK GENERATOR

It has long been known that the refuse "slop" from whiskey distillers greatly increases the quantity of milk from cows. This has been found to be due to the large amounts of yeast it contains. It's upon the same principle that both ale and porter have earned such a great reputation as milk generators. From the ancient Greeks on down, all authors on this subject recommend fermented grain beverages. Many nursing women in Ireland drink the dark Guinness stout beer, which is rich in yeast and therefore rich in B vitamins. But be sure when using beer, and particularly porter, to avoid excess, because if taken too copiously it will eventually reduce milk production, and eventually entirely eliminate it. With all such alcoholic beverages, moderation must always be the watchword.

A particularly fine combination consists of two or three parts cow's milk with one part Guinness stout or other additive-free beer. This combination is a bit less stimulating to the mother and more nourishing than beer by itself, and it often aids in increasing the pleasure of nursing.

Regarding wine: again, a glass or two, especially of higher quality wines that are free of additives (if they can be found), may not increase the flow of milk but may be of benefit in relaxing the mother.

TIME-TESTED RECIPES GIVEN

A recipe published in London in 1596 is reproduced here, again for historical purposes:

A very good medicine to increase milk in a woman's breasts. Take fennel roots and parsnip roots and let them be boiled in broth which must be made of chickens. Then let the patient eat the same roots with fresh butter, which must be new made as possibly it may be gotten, and this will cause great store of milk to increase in any woman's breasts. This has been often proved.

Another recipe is:

Take rice and sieve it in cow's milk and cream some wheaten bread therein; it must be such as clean without rye, and put into the said milk some fennel seed beaten into fine powder and a little sugar to make it sweet, and this is known to be exceedingly good.

HERBAL PROMOTERS OF HUMAN MILK

Herbs. Herbal galactagogues, or promoters of milk flow, are rarely recommended to nursing mothers today, not because they may be harmful but rather because galactagogues are not usually described in herbal books and are certainly not discussed in medical schools, and so many doctors neither know of nor believe in their existence. We list here those plants that have been found to be most efficacious and are most frequently named by both ancient and relatively recent authorities in the world of herbal medicine.

Borage: The seeds and leaves are used.

Common lettuce: Particularly the juice is used.

Rocket (Eruca sativa): This plant, which is known in southern Europe, was discussed by Culpepper, who said: "The seed also taken in drink taketh away the ill scent from the arm-pits, increaseth milk in nurses, and wasteth the spleen." The eleventh-century physician Avicenna states that there are two varieties, a cultivated and a wild one. He claims that the milk is increased when the seed is boiled into a decoction and put on instead of mustard as a poultice.

Cassava or *Manioc:* This is commonly known as "tapioca," whose meal is mixed with as much boiling water as it will absorb and in this state is eaten as ordinary porridge. It should be pointed out, though, that this plant is simply rich in carbohydrates and is a very poor source of nitrogen or proteins.

Wintergreen (Gualtheria procumbens): This plant is listed here *not* as a recommended galactagogue but *to be avoided.* While it is perfectly safe for nonpregnant women and particularly enjoyed for its aromatic qualities, a death has been reported from the use of wintergreen oil, and it should be avoided by all means.

Basil: This is another ancient galactagogue, and may simply be used as a spice.

Milk vetch: This herb when taken as a decoction is said to increase milk and has been used as such for centuries. This plant was formerly kept by herbalists for suckling mothers specifically, and was also known as "milkweed." It is second only to fennel and quite readily available in herb stores. The leaves are simply made up as a tea.

Marshmallow (Malva sylvestris): "The leaves boiled used by nurses procureth them abundance of milk" (Culpepper). A variety of *Malva* was spoken of as long ago as in the time of Avicenna under the name of *cubeze,* "which is a wild kind of Malva, as the Mulochia is a domestic variety." The leaves and flowers were used to improve the flow of milk.

Lastly, there are several plants, members of the *Umbelliferae,* which have been highly recommended since antiquity. These include *anise, fennel, parsley,* and the *carrot.* All of these plants are certainly too well known to require description, and ancient authors from Hippocrates onward speak of them as excellent aids in promoting the secretion of milk.

STROKING AND JOKING GOOD FOR NURSING MOTHER

Environmental and Emotional Factors. Although improved diet and use of herbs alone may be sufficient to correct a decreased flow of milk and to improve its quality, there are other factors that can reduce milk flow, and these must also be considered. Certainly you must avoid states of fear and other violent emotions. Excessive obesity may have a detrimental effect, as can poor air in the mother's environment. Finally, the relationship between husband and wife is especially important during this period. The husband should participate to some extent in nursing the child by demonstrating his affection and tenderness toward both infant and mother. In fact, it has long been found that a woman who shares actively moments of tenderness with her mate during the period of nursing tends to have a more successful, problem-free nursing experience.

WEANING

Changing Patterns of Weaning

WEANING DEFINED

Weaning has been variously defined as the cessation of breast-feeding, the introduction of foods other than breast milk, or a combination of the two. Among the ancients the weaning period generally coincided with the period of teething, with new foods being gradually introduced and nursing gradually decreasing and finally ending about the time when the last milk teeth appeared.

BREAD DIPPED IN WINE

The ancient Greeks generally began weaning at about six months, at the time the teeth usually began to appear, introducing bread crumbs soaked in fluids such as water, sweetened milk, wine, bone, or vegetable broth. The Bible mentions a weaning food of corn and wine. For the ancients these added foods were of relatively minor importance; in fact, milk teeth were so named because during the period when they appeared, breast milk was the principal food and very little other food was added. At the completion of weaning the child was considered able to eat anything, although breast-feeding might be resumed if the child became ill.

Weaning was generally completed no earlier than the age of two years, an age favored not only by the Greeks but also by the Bible and the Koran. Spring and autumn were preferred for weaning, and summer weaning was discouraged because it was often accompanied by diarrhea or other problems. The ancients further expressed a preference for weaning during the waxing moon.

WEANING CEREMONIES

The termination of nursing was often celebrated among the Greeks by public weaning ceremonies, where a bad-tasting substance like pepper or mustard would be smeared on the mother's nipple and the breast offered to the unsuspecting child, whose surprise and displeasure would greatly amuse the onlookers. The breast might be offered and refused a second time, and weaning was complete.

WEANING TIME NOW EARLIER

Over the ensuing centuries there has been a general tendency for the period of nursing to become shorter, with weaning being completed well before the last appearance of teeth. Eventually many people theorized that prolonged nursing was bad for the child. More recently, weaning has been initiated before the onset of teething. Present practice is often to begin both cereal and noncereal foods before the age of six months, at earlier and earlier ages.

When and How to Begin Solid Foods

BLENDERIZED FOODS ADVISED

What is the proper time for weaning? There is no specific rule for this, but at some point your nursing infant must be given solid food. If the mother has been properly nourished during pregnancy, there is no reason why solid food must be begun before the age of six months. It could be begun a little sooner or a little later, but preferably not before four months of age. Feeding at this time is a supplement to the mother's milk, and a chief problem to overcome is a mechanical one: namely, the infant's difficulty with chewing. It's extremely simple to puree in a blender some of the same food the rest of your family eats and give this to your baby. By using a home blender you need not prepare or purchase special "baby foods."

FOOD SAME AS FOR REST OF FAMILY

By the time your baby is about six months old, he or she can eat almost any soft blenderized food. We recommend that your child be given in a blenderized form much the same food as the rest of the family so that from an early age he can become accustomed to eating table foods.

PROTEIN QUALITY EMPHASIZED

What sorts of foods should be added? Very often you will hear that young babies need a very high protein diet. This is a myth. The proper proportion of protein to total calories, or the density of protein, in a child's diet is really little different from that required by an adult. What *is* really important is that the so-called protein quality— that is, the relative amount of essential amino acids found in the food—must be higher in an infant's or child's food than in an adult's. During this period, high-quality protein foods (containing all essential amino acids) that are derived from *animal* sources, such as milk products, eggs, and small amounts of meat, fish, or poultry without skin, should be served in addition to the regular diet of the family. If you are vegetarian, mix complementary grains and legumes (such as corn and beans) to provide a complete complement of the essential amino acids, and be sure to include egg and dairy foods in your baby's diet as well.

You can continue to breast-feed until the child is

about two years of age, as is still done in most of the less technologically developed world. In our society, in which many mothers want to return to the workplace, this can be very inconvenient; and breast-feeding for about eight months or a year is certainly sufficient to ensure the adequate nutrition of the child and the formation of a bond between you and your baby. By this time your child can often drink from a cup with the family and begin to munch on various types of solid foods without much difficulty.

After weaning, the child can eat much the same food as an adult does, but high-quality protein should be pres-

TABLE 3
Foods Added to the Infant's Diet

Age	Foods
Birth through 12th month	Human milk or formula (iron fortified), or evaporated milk (+ supplemental vitamin/ mineral formula)
4th through 6th months	ADD dry-type infant cereal (no sugar or preservatives) (+ vit/min)
4th through 7th months	ADD vegetables, fruits, and their juices (squeezed or blenderized) (+ vit/min)
6th through 8th months	ADD egg yolk, meat, fish, poultry without skin, well-cooked beans, yogurt, and cheese (+ vit/min)
10th through 12th months	ADD whole egg (+ vit/min)

ent in adequate amounts. By about age four, an adult diet, as outlined in Book II, is appropriate. The preceding table summarizes which foods should be introduced from birth through the twelfth month. Bear in mind, please, that this is a sequential recommendation for the introduction of solid foods; that is, the foods added at higher age levels are in addition to the foods that preceded them, so that by age twelve months all of the foods in the right column will be part of an infant's diet. Remember also that vitamin and mineral supplementation will probably be required in most infant diets, and the nutrients most likely to be in short supply in breast milk or in formula are vitamin A, iron, vitamin D, and folic acid.

Prepared Baby Foods

WHAT'S IN BABY FOODS?

If you choose to use prepared baby foods, you need to use your best detective skills to figure out exact nutritional information regarding many commercially prepared foods. One way you can learn just what they contain is to purchase a copy of the 1978 U.S. Department of Agriculture Handbook 8–3, which shows the amino-acid and fatty-acid content of most commercially prepared baby foods. If you're worried about additives, lactose intolerance, or food allergies, we suggest that you write directly to the three principal baby-food companies and ask them for detailed information on the exact ingredients of specific products. Their addresses are: Beech-Nut Corporation, Fort Washington, Pa. 19034; Gerber Products Company, 445 State Street, Fremont, Mi. 49412; Heinz, P.O. Box 57, Pittsburgh, Pa. 15230. The present trend is for these three companies to reduce or eliminate completely sugar from baby foods. Another trend is toward excluding salt, particularly sodium, from these products.

Sodium in Your Baby's Food

SOME SALT NECESSARY

There is still a question as to whether a high intake of sodium during infancy predisposes the child to develop high blood pressure later on when he is an adult. Evidence shows that there is a strong relationship between high sodium intake and increased blood-pressure levels in adults; yet we have no way of knowing whether adding salt to infant foods is harmful. The taste for salt is definitely an acquired one, and we should tend to diminish the amount of sodium in our babies' diets, to discourage excessive desire for salt, *but should not exclude it entirely.*

An infant needs only a very little bit of sodium each day. In the 1980 RDAs, safe intake for sodium is 115–350 mg. from birth through the sixth month, and 250–750 mg. from the sixth month to the first year. Cow's milk contains about three times as much sodium as does human milk, while skim milk contains almost nine times as much sodium, owing to its concentration. As solid foods are added to your baby's diet, sodium levels also increase, since sodium occurs naturally in most foods. You should remember that homemade baby foods made from your table meals very often contain *more* sodium than commercial baby foods, particularly if salt-rich foods and seasonings are used by your family.

Why to Avoid Canned Foods

CANNED FOODS MAY CONTAIN LEAD AND TIN

We advise you not to feed infants canned foods. Unless they are specifically packaged for infants and labeled as such, canned fruits and vegetables are to be avoided because the amount of salt in canned vegetables is usually high, and the heavy syrup in canned fruits contains a large amount of sugar. Another problem is that canned foods often contain low levels of lead, which is an extremely dangerous metal, especially for the young. Many infant formulas are made with evaporated milk. An often overlooked contaminant of canned evaporated milk is tin. The tin content of such milk was found to increase linearly with storage time. West African children given one six-ounce can of such milk that had been stored for six months were found to be taking in 12.5 mg. of tin, and only 4.5 mg. is considered "safe" for an adult!

Encourage Use of a Cup

NO SWEETS IN THAT BOTTLE!

Avoid putting your baby to bed with a nursing bottle that contains fruit juice or water with some sugar or honey. Decay-producing bacteria grow well in such sweet substances and can begin their work of destroying your baby's teeth. This is why we recommend that you teach your baby to drink from a cup as soon after the sixth month as possible, and that use of bottles be discouraged. Bedtime bottles of fruit juice, milk, or Jell-O water are unnecessary once teeth have appeared. If she insists on a bottle, make sure it contains purified water only. By all means say no to sodas, fruit drinks, and other heavily sweetened liquids.

Skim and Low-Fat Milk: Not for Infants

FULL-FAT MILK ADVISED

Should we give our babies skim and low-fat milk? Low-fat diets for adults are now very popular in America because it is believed that such diets discourage the development of atherosclerosis and also may reduce the incidence of some cancers. As a result, many concerned parents are increasingly using nonfat or low-fat milk for feeding their infants. It's important that this practice be discontinued. Not only is the evidence scanty that low-fat diets prevent the development of heart disease, but in some cases they can have harmful effects on your baby.

What happens is this. Babies who are given skim milk exclusively drink *more* in an attempt to make up for the lower amount of calories. By having to drink a greater volume of milk to be satisfied, your child is being conditioned to having to eat more in order to be satisfied, and you could be setting the stage for the development of obesity later in life. Secondly, because skim milk has a higher relative-protein content and a greater electrolyte content, an added burden is placed on the infant's kidneys, which can be hazardous to babies with conditions, such as diarrhea, related to increased loss of fluids.

While low-fat milk contains about 2 percent fat and has some dry milk solids added, it is really not much better. In any case, skim milk should *never* be used as the only infant food, because it lacks necessary fat and contains excessive quantities of other nutrients. It is also devoid of linoleic acid, which is not found in nonfat milk. This essential fatty acid, in conjunction with other nutrients, namely vitamins C and B_6 and zinc, is needed to help stimulate the immune system.

FAT NEEDED FOR CALCIUM ABSORPTION

Another good reason for feeding whole milk to babies is that in order for calcium to be properly absorbed, fat is definitely necessary in the milk, particularly during the calcium-sensitive time of infancy.

Of course, for babies with a tendency toward high levels of cholesterol, the intake of fat, from cow's milk and human milk alike, must be limited. For the normal baby without such a disorder, however, we do not recommend the use of skim or low fat milk, especially on an exclusive basis.

BOOK II
The Diet of Older Children

TEACHING GOOD NUTRITION

SCHOOL-AGE CHILDREN SELECT OWN FOODS

Your child's growth takes place in a series of spurts, alternating with periods of slower growth, up through the end of adolescence (see Figure 1). Throughout this period, sound nutrition is essential. The dietary advice in Book I will see you and your baby through the critical periods of pregnancy, infancy, and the preschool years, but when your youngster is ready to leave the environment of the home to attend school, it is particularly important to instill in him an understanding of proper nutrition, since he will be making dietary decisions on his own that can have far-reaching consequences for his growth and development.

PERSONALITY CHANGES FROM JUNK FOOD

Unfortunately, many of our children are making the wrong decisions about what to eat. A recent study at the Cleveland Medical Center identified a form of malnutrition among adolescents who ate large quantities of junk food, to the neglect of essential elements of the diet. The

FIGURE 1
Growth Cycles—Birth to Maturity*

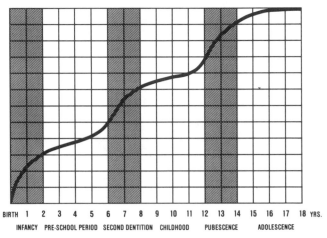

From birth to maturity growth is continuous, but falls into three cycles. Growth is rapid in infancy, and then slows during the preschool years; growth is again rapid during the period of second dentition, and is slower during childhood; and the rapid growth during pubescence is followed by the slower growth of adolescence.

*After Dr. I.N. Kugelmass (1946).

resulting deficiency of thiamin (vitamin B_1), somewhat resembling the classic deficiency disease beriberi, produced symptoms such as severe personality changes including aggressive behavior and irritability, as well as abdominal and chest pains, restlessness, insomnia, and bad dreams.

SIMPLE EATING GUIDELINES GIVEN

Good nutrition for children is not particularly complicated or mysterious. In a letter distributed to parents, the innovative Castlemont School of Encino, California, outlined the following simple ideas as the basis of its highly successful nutritional awareness program:

Castlemont Guidelines for Lunches*

TO EAT:

Include foods from the four basic food groups:
a. Fruits and vegetables   c. Milk products
b. Grains, cereals   d. Meat, chicken, fish, nuts

SANDWICH IDEAS:

a. Beef (without nitrates)   g. Hard boiled egg
b. Chicken   h. Peanut butter (pure,
c. Turkey   not hydrogenated)
d. Cheese (natural)   i. Fruit and nut butters
e. Tuna   such as apple,
f. Egg salad   strawberry, etc.

RAW VEGETABLES

a. Carrot strips   g. Green-pepper strips
b. Celery sticks   h. Jicama strips
c. Radishes   i. Turnip strips
d. Cauliflower florets   j. Sprouts, bean or alfalfa
e. Cucumber strips   k. Lettuce
f. Cherry tomatoes

FRUITS: DRIED FRUIT:

a. Apples   g. Strawberries   a. Apricots
b. Bananas   h. Oranges   b. Dates
c. Cherries   i. Tangerines   c. Figs
d. Grapes   j. Pineapple   d. Prunes
e. Peaches   k. Pomegranate   e. Raisins
f. Plums   l. Pears

NUTRITIOUS TREATS:

a. Raw nuts: almonds, cashews, pecans, walnuts, filberts, etc.
b. Granola
c. Crackers with natural ingredients
d. Seeds: pumpkin, sesame, sunflower, etc.
e. Homemade breads and cakes (date, zucchini, carrot, apple, pumpkin)
f. Homemade pretzels (unsalted)
g. Graham crackers (without preservatives)
h. Trail mix
i. Peanut-butter balls (honey, peanut butter, noninstant dry milk)

TO DRINK:

a. Milk—any kind
b. Pure juices: apple, grape, pineapple, orange, etc.

FOODS NOT ALLOWED AT SCHOOL:

a. Candy
b. Soda pop
c. Beverages in cans marked "punch" or "drink"
d. Desserts that fall in the category of sticky cakes, doughnuts, and rich pastries

*From Kathy Craft, "Castlemont School—Where Nutrition Is a Way of Life," *Let's Live*, August 1979, pp. 42–47.

CHILDREN OFTEN COOPERATE IN DIETARY REFORM

It might surprise you how readily a well-informed child can learn to give up a junk-food habit and adopt good eating practices, once the reasons are presented clearly. The experience of the Castlemont School demonstrates that children *can* learn to prefer the foods that are good for them. In this chapter we will review the nutritional considerations that must go into the makeup of each of your child's daily meals, showing the rationale behind such simple eating plans as the Castlemont program. Of course, it is of the utmost importance that you be able to offer tasty alternatives to dangerous junk foods, and for this purpose we provide a wide selection of healthful and palatable recipes in Book IV.

How to Avoid Contaminants in Foods

MANY DANGERS IN COMMON FOODS

Not only dietary deficiencies but also the additives and contaminants in our foods can jeopardize our youngsters' health. We must be constantly on guard against such artificial substances as food colorings, flavorings, and preservatives, so many of which have been shown to produce allergic reactions in some individuals, as well as being highly suspect as cancer-causing agents.

From the discussion that follows, it may sometimes appear that it is a hopeless struggle to try to assure the safety of our children's food supply. But alternatives *do* exist. It *is* possible to ensure an adequate, nutritious, and palatable diet for our youngsters, while at the same time avoiding the many artificial ingredients, additives, and other contaminants that are so widely used in the food industry today.

MUCH INFORMATION ON FOOD LABELS

The first step is to learn how to read the labels on any packaged foods you buy. Ingredients are listed in order according to their percentage by weight in the product. Thus the first ingredient listed is the one present in the greatest quantity, and the last one in the smallest quantity. Once you know this, you will discover that many supposedly nutritious foods consist mainly of water and sugar, with the "natural" ingredients proclaimed on the package actually proving to fall far down on the list! Of course, the label must also list all preservatives, artificial colorings, and flavorings, and will reveal the presence of salt and unsuspected sugar in the form of added dextrose, fructose, or sucrose.

A 1975 regulation, which food manufacturers may observe on an optional basis, calls for additional information on the labels of some foods, including an analysis of nutrients on a per-serving basis; the caloric content of the food as well as the protein, carbohydrate, and fat content in grams; protein content expressed as a percentage of the RDA; the content of at least seven vitamins and minerals; and an optional listing of cholesterol, fatty-acid, and sodium content. By learning to look for and evaluate this information on food packages, you can invest your food dollars much more wisely when you shop, and protect your family's health at the same time.

COOKING FROM SCRATCH ADVISED

Another solution, of course, is to avoid processed foods and cook more of your meals from scratch. The recipes in Book IV will help to free you of overreliance on many processed foods (such as breakfast cereals) and to develop meal plans around dishes whose wholesomeness is guaranteed because you know exactly what is in them!

BREAKFAST

Better is a dry morsel and quietness therewith
than a house full of feasting with strife.
                    PROVERBS 17:1

COMPONENTS OF AN ADEQUATE BREAKFAST OUTLINED

Of all meals breakfast is king. Without adequate levels of protein, fat, a slow-burning carbohydrate fuel, and adequate amounts of vitamins and minerals, your child will lack concentration in school and be more susceptible to colds and other childhood complaints. Instead of looking forward to each day, your youngster may just go through the paces without really caring.

VITAMIN PILLS NOT ENOUGH

A vitamin pill does not magically turn the average glass of juice and sweetened, cold cereal with milk into a good breakfast. That pill is *never* a substitute for good food, only a supplement. In fact, in my experience, vitamins fail to be effective unless taken with a good, substantial meal.

Let's take a look at those breakfast cereals and cottony white breads that occupy such a prominent place on the supermarket shelves. To understand why these products may not be the nourishing foods their manufacturers claim they are, we'll need to understand what has happened to the grains from which they're made, before they arrive on your breakfast table.

Grains—the Universal Staple

WHEAT AND RICE WORLD'S LEADING FOODS

Grains are an extremely important food worldwide, providing about 80 percent of the world's food calories and covering about 70 percent of the cultivated land on our planet. The biggest grain crop is wheat; but rice, which covers considerably less of the world's grain-growing acreage, is used by more people as their chief food. Other common grains include oats, corn, barley, rye, and the less familiar buckwheat and millet. Each of these grains is an important staple food for people somewhere in the world.

WHOLE GRAINS RICH IN NUTRIENTS

In their natural, unprocessed form, whole grains are an important source of nutrients, including vitamin E, many of the B vitamins, iron, and protein. Since they also contain up to 60 percent starch, they are a significant source of caloric energy as well. The proteins in grains are not complete proteins; that is, they do *not* supply all the essential amino acids needed for proper bodily function, and so many ethnic recipes wisely combine grains with other foods to provide the complete protein our bodies require. As a general rule, it's a good idea to combine grains in the diet with complete protein foods such as meat, eggs, and milk to ensure a proper supply of the amino acids needed for building and rebuilding active bodies.

STONE-GRINDING YIELDS HEALTHFUL FLOUR

Breads. Although all grains are used to some extent in their whole, unprocessed form to make cooked cereal foods, by far the most common way of preparing grains for the past 2000 years has been to grind them into flour. The local gristmill used to be an important part of village life. Using grinding stones, the miller would break up the kernels of grains such as wheat, corn, and rye to make nutritious whole-grain flours. In this stone-grinding process the cellular structure of the grain is not greatly disturbed, and the nutritious germ of the grain and the bran are retained. This whole-grain flour could then be made into a wide variety of healthful baked goods, including the dark, substantial whole-grain breads our ancestors valued so highly as the "staff of life."

WHITE FLOUR ROBBED OF NUTRIENTS

A couple of centuries ago, it became fashionable to use a lighter-colored flour to make cakes and pastry. The darker, whole-grain flour came to be considered "poor people's food," while the white flour, which had become whiter because most of its nutritious elements had been removed, was supposedly more suitable for the wealthy. With the introduction of large-scale steel-milling after the American Civil War, grain was no longer ground but was instead crushed, flattening out the germ and the bran in the process. When the flour was sifted, these elements of the grain, which contain most of the fiber, B vitamins and minerals, all the vitamin E, and a large amount of the higher-quality protein, were discarded. The resultant product was a white, starchy, powdery kind of flour with very little nutritional value.

For an idea of what is lost when the wheat grain is milled into white flour, Table 4, which follows, will be helpful. Note that upward of 86 percent of some nutrients are lost in milling.

WHEAT GERM A GOOD FOOD

It is an irony of modern food technology that the food processors frequently remove the nutrients from whole, fresh foods, only to sell these nutrients back to us as dietary supplements, at greatly increased prices! Nevertheless, it is worthwhile to invest in wheat germ as a supplement to your child's diet. If she doesn't like the taste of wheat germ by itself, you can sprinkle it on her breakfast cereal, or on ice cream, applesauce, or other desserts, lending a nutty, crunchy flavor that is supercharged nutritionally. The wheat germ sold in the supermarket is not of as high a quality as untoasted varieties available in some health-food stores, since most of the vitamin E and essential oils are missing in the commercial brands, but even these products are better than no wheat germ at all.

Although some of the germ and bran removed from our grain find their way into cereals and supplements, much more of these nutritious products is used for animal feed. It seems that people who raise livestock are

TABLE 4
A Comparison of Whole Wheat
Versus White Flour*

Nutrient	Whole Wheat mcg/gm	White Flour mcg/gm	Loss in Refining %
Thiamine	3.5	0.8	77.1
Riboflavin	1.5	0.3	80.0
Niacin	50	9.5	80.8
Vitamin B₆	1.7	0.5	71.8
Pantothenic acid	10	5	50.0
Folacin	0.3	0.1	66.7
α-Tocopherol	16	2.2	86.3
Choline	1089	767	29.5
Manganese	46	6.5	85.8
Iron	43	10.5	75.6
Zinc	35	7.8	77.7
	%	%	
Calcium	0.045	0.018	60.0
Phosphorus	0.433	0.126	70.9
Magnesium	0.183	0.028	84.7
Potassium	0.454	0.105	77.0

*After Briggs and Calloway (1979).

more aware of the value of germ and bran in their animals' feed than the food manufacturers are of their importance in the human diet!

SHELF LIFE FAVORED OVER HUMAN LIFE

But why should nonnutritious white flour be so popular today? The main reason is that our all-powerful food-processing industry knows that this white flour is easier to store for long periods of time. Because the bran and germ have been removed, bacteria and insects cannot live on stored white flour. Moreover, the germ contains essential oils that will eventually turn rancid in whole-grain flour unless it is refrigerated. It is therefore less expensive to store grain in the form of white flour. Commercial baked-goods manufacturers can also produce bread and other products using this flour, which will have a longer shelf life, resulting in fewer costly returns of stale goods.

Our criticism of white flour is not purely theoretical. There is historical and epidemiological evidence that white flour is not good for us, based on the experience of populations in wartime who weren't able to get the highly milled flours to which they had become accustomed. In Denmark during World War I, for example, the nutritional status of the population actually *improved* when they were not able to obtain milled flour; their food supply otherwise remained largely the same as before the war, since Denmark's agriculture was able to provide the country's food needs.

"ENRICHED" FLOUR A MISNOMER

What about the "enriched" white flours that are sold today and the breads made from such flours? Let's remember that this flour started as nutritious, whole grains, from which the refining process removed most of the higher-quality protein, iron, other minerals, B vitamins, and vitamin E. To enrich the flour, three B vitamins—thiamine, riboflavin, and niacin—are put back in; it is no coincidence that these happen to be the cheapest of all the vitamins. Some iron is also added, and sometimes calcium and vitamin D. These nutrients are added in smaller quantities than were originally present in the grain; but missing forever are the vitamin E, the other B vitamins, zinc, selenium, fiber, and other important nutrients once supplied by man's ancient "staff of life," which is now little more than a feeble crutch.

But that's not the end of the story. White flour is also

bleached with chlorine dioxide, destroying any vitamin E that may remain after milling. Experiments have shown that flour treated with chlorine dioxide will stunt the growth of mice to which it is fed. In addition, many questionable chemicals are added to the bleached, starchy powder that is today's sorry version of flour, including softeners, fresheners, mold inhibitors, and aging ingredients.

This is a pretty frightening picture of what lurks in a loaf of white bread. And yet many people have been so taken in by advertising and the ever-present trickery inducing them to buy these devitalized grain products that they actually think white bread tastes better than whole-grain bread. But there are alternatives, and we owe it to our children's health to provide them with nutritious, whole-grain breads, made from stone-ground grains, and to protect them from the harmful additives and valueless ingredients in our popular white breads.

FLOUR LABELS DEMYSTIFIED

First, a caution, which will be emphasized repeatedly throughout this book. *We must be very critical when we read the labels on processed foods.* As we have just seen, "enriched" flour isn't as rich as the grain from which it was made. Another example is the so-called wheat flour or "unbleached wheat flour" referred to on packages of flour and bread. This should not be confused with whole-wheat flour; *by FDA standards, wheat flour and unbleached wheat flour are the same as white flour!* Even cracked-wheat and rye breads may really be white bread dyed with caramel coloring.

GOOD BREAD DOES EXIST

Fortunately, thanks to the growth of conscientious independent bakeries in recent years, you *can* find nutritious stone-ground whole-grain breads today at reputable health-food stores, and even some of the larger super-markets are now carrying these products. You will find many interesting combinations of whole grains in these substantial, satisfying loaves, with a wide range of flavors and textures that will provide your child with a new ap-preciation for this age-old staple food.

MARGARINE, SUGAR, TO BE AVOIDED

What to spread on bread? In later sections of this chapter we'll discuss what may be spread on this tasty whole-grain bread. For your child's health, butter must always be preferred over margarine, owing to the chemi-cals and hydrogenated oils in the cheaper spread; and if sweet jams, jellies, and fruit butters are to be eaten, be sure they are made from fruit and perhaps a little honey. We'll be taking a closer look at fruit preserves when we talk about some ideas for lunch.

Pancakes and waffles. Pancakes and waffles are also good breakfast foods, but be sure these are also the whole-grain variety. You will find a highly nutritious waf-fle recipe in Book IV under "Breakfast" entries. And re-member, pancake syrup must be pure, not just some corn sweetener with added artificial flavoring.

BREAKFAST CEREALS HIGH IN PROFITS, LOW IN NUTRIENTS

Breakfast cereals. Cereals are defined as grains con-sumed by humans; the term should conjure up images of fields of golden wheat, its heavy heads swaying in the breeze. The contents of most of the cereal packages on our supermarket shelves are but a faint shadow of this wholesome picture, however. The food industry has dis-covered that it can produce dry breakfast cereals very cheaply and sell them at a very high price, increasing their profits tremendously. These breakfast cereals may contain little more than carbohydrates, since they are produced from devitalized, overly processed grains. With the help of multimillion-dollar advertising campaigns, these products are foisted on the public as alleged sources of valuable nutrients and energy. Yet experiments have shown that laboratory animals fed on breakfast cereals alone have suffered retarded growth!

To counter this problem, the "Breakfast" recipes contained in Book IV are all made with high-quality grains, yet are easily prepared. See especially the "Weimar Kitchen" recipes for almond-crunch granola, cashew French toast, granola pudding, and the mixed-grain waffles. The note on "How to Cook Cereals" will be very helpful.

MUCH SUGAR IN PACKAGED CEREALS

Of course, the worst thing done to breakfast cereals is the addition of sucrose and other cheap sweeteners. Some cereals actually contain more sugar than grain, as you will discover when you study the labels. In an insidious advertising campaign aimed directly at our children (cereal manufacturers spent $186 million on advertising in 1978), favorite cartoon characters and television personalities exhort their kiddie audiences to eat these sugary breakfast foods. Through the eating of these products, children develop an acquired craving for more and more sugar, for excessive sweetness in all their food.

In a recent analysis of 62 brands of breakfast cereal, published by the U.S. Department of Agriculture, it was shown that the sugar content may run as high as 56 percent. Even brands without obvious sugar coating may contain significant amounts of added sugar. There is an interesting correlation between the amount spent on advertising a particular cereal and its sugar content; apparently, Americans are not particularly eager to buy the highly sugared brands without considerable encouragement. In fact, several highly sugared brands have gone off the market in recent years, while cereals with little or no added sugar remain perennial favorites.

WHOLE-GRAIN CEREALS ADVISED

As with breads, there *is* a way out of this terrifying maze of corporate manipulation of our children's diet. Even in the supermarket, there are some products, such as steel-cut oats and whole-grain hot cereals (great with cottage cheese!), that will provide proper nutrition at the breakfast table. By carefully reading the labels on cereals, you will be able to find some that contain grains that have not been overly processed and sweetened to death. Of course, you can also make cooked cereals from whole grains purchased in bulk at a health-food store; the section "How to Cook Cereals" in Book IV will tell you how.

GRANOLA MAY BE HIGHLY SUGARED

What about granola? Many nutritious granolas, made of whole grains such as oats mixed with dried fruits, nuts, and other healthful foods, are available on the market today. Unfortunately, almost all of these granolas contain added sweetening, and we should be alert to avoid those sweetened with refined sugar, or with excessive quantities of *any* sweetener, including honey. Of the 14 commercially produced granolas analyzed in a USDA study, sugar content ranged from 22 to 31 percent, usually in the form of sucrose. It is a good idea to buy your granola in a health-food store, where it may be available in bulk, but be sure to inquire about added sweeteners. The surest way to avoid added sugar is to make your own granola, using the granola recipes in

Book IV, which rely on the natural sweetness of dates and other dried fruits rather than on added sweetener of any kind.

Milk. The milk poured on your child's breakfast cereal, as well as that in a tall glass, is an important part of the start of every day for most children. In our discussion of foods for lunch, we will be talking about the role of milk and other dairy products in the diet.

Eggs

EGGS A GOOD FOOD FOR MOST CHILDREN

A favorite breakfast food for many children, eggs are an excellent way to start off the day with a good source of complete protein. They also supply iron and vitamins A and D and riboflavin.

As Americans are becoming increasingly aware, egg yolks are also a source of cholesterol, and many adults are avoiding eggs in their diet. Although such advisory bodies as the Senate Select Committee on Human Nutrition have advised a general reduction of cholesterol intake in the diet, this does not generally apply to normal, healthy children, who are able to metabolize normal quantities of cholesterol in their food. However, there are certain genetic conditions that may be present in families, such as hyperlipoproteinemia. These families should avoid the excessive eating of eggs even among children.

MANY EGGS PRODUCED UNNATURALLY

Although they are a very rich source of nutrients, eggs are produced under less than ideal circumstances in today's food industry. The chickens live under highly artificial conditions, cooped up in cages with no room to move around, living under artificial light and in controlled temperatures, and fed by automatic equipment. Of course, these birds would be living much closer to their natural state if they were allowed to run loose and peck at wholesome grain growing in the soil, and the unnatural conditions under which they are raised must have an effect on the quality of their eggs.

ORGANIC EGGS ADVISED

Even worse, assembly-line chicken farms add a large number of chemicals to the chickens' feed, including antibiotics, hormones, pesticides, and tranquilizers— each designed to increase egg production with little concern for the well-being of the chickens, which have been turned into nothing more than biological egg-producing machines. All these chemicals pass directly through the chicken into the egg. It is possible to avoid these potentially harmful contaminants by buying "organically grown" eggs at health-food stores or other reputable markets. The labeling on the cartons will tell you whether you are getting eggs that have been produced from chickens without using adulterants and drugs.

Incidentally, there is no nutritional difference between brown and white eggs; the color simply comes from the breed of hen that laid them.

Breakfast Meats: A Warning on Nitrites

SALTING MEATS AN ANCIENT PRACTICE

As a favorite accompaniment to eggs at breakfast, many families regularly eat such preserved meats as bacon, ham, and sausage. The practice of preserving meats is nearly as old as the eating of meat itself. From earliest times man has known that meat and fish could be kept from spoiling by adding salt, which hastened the drying process and retarded the growth of harmful molds and bacteria. In more recent times it was found that a different salt, sodium nitrite, would turn patches of meat red, and so modern meat processors use sodium nitrite in the curing of meats such as bacon and ham to prevent them from turning an unappealing grayish-brown color. These preservatives also inhibit the growth of dangerous bacteria such as those that cause botulism.

NITRITES AND NITRATES DANGEROUS

Unfortunately, there is ever-increasing evidence that nitrites are very dangerous to our health. In the stomach these salts are converted to nitrous acid, which apparently interferes with the genetic material in living cells, and has been shown to produce mutations in the cells of many lower organisms. Because of its suspected ability to cause mutations in cells, nitrous acid may, it is thought, produce stomach cancer in humans. This same nitrous acid may also react in the digestive tract with amines derived from other foods to produce nitrosamines, which are violent carcinogens, especially in children.

For the same reasons, we should be suspicious of nitrates in our foods. Although nitrates are relatively harmless themselves, bacteria in the stomach convert them into nitrites—especially in children, who have a higher concentration of bacteria in their stomachs, enabling the nitrates to be broken down more readily.

VITAMIN C A SAFE PRESERVATIVE

Recognizing the potential dangers of nitrites and nitrates, a number of countries have banned or severely limited the use of these substances in foods. Certainly there are other ways of preserving color in meats; vitamin C, for example, is an excellent substitute.

READ LABELS ON CURED MEATS

Despite the reluctance of regulatory agencies in this country to make a move against nitrites and nitrates in our food, we must take the initiative in protecting our children's health and check the labels of all cured meats—sausage, ham, bacon, bologna, hot dogs, smoked fish, and the like—and *avoid any preserved foods that contain these dangerous substances.*

Fruits and Juices

Breakfast should also include fruit or juice, which is discussed in detail in the section that follows.

MID-MORNING SNACKS

ALTERNATIVES TO JUNK FOODS IMPERATIVE

With their high expenditure of energy, children are usually eager for a snack by mid-morning, and again in midafternoon. If we are careful to provide them with healthful, nourishing treats, they will be less likely to resort to the gooey, sugary, mass-produced pastries, the greasy potato chips, the tooth-demolishing candies and sodas, that are all too available outside the home. An excellent choice for mid-morning is a piece of fresh, ripe fruit; other possibilities are discussed under "Midafternoon Snacks," and delicious recipes are found under "Sweet Things" in Book IV.

Fruits

DATES A DESSERT STAPLE

Because of their natural sweetness and their nutritional value, fruits have been an important element of the human diet for a very long time; many fruits familiar today have been cultivated for thousands of years. In some cultures, wise and efficient use of fruits has made them into dietary staples. The date, for example, often serves as the principal or sole food of certain Arab tribes who live in areas where food supplies are often unreliable. Eaten fresh or dried, preserved by boiling in salted water, and even made into long-keeping flour, as well as honey and wine, dates have proved extremely versatile for these desert dwellers. Although dates consist largely of sugar, with only 2 percent each of protein and fat, these tribal peoples generally eat them with milk, yogurt, or cheese, and this combination provides a diet that will sustain life for long periods of time.

LONG-LIVED HUNZA FAVOR VERSATILE APRICOT

The Hunza people of the Himalayas, fabled for their longevity, make similar use of apricots, which they eat fresh in season and then dry for storage. The apricot kernels are eaten, stored as nuts, and used as a source of oil. Proponents of the anticancer drug laetrile, which is derived from the kernels of fruits such as apricots, speculate that perhaps it is the eating of these kernels that may account for the reputed nonexistence of cancer among the Hunza.

FRUIT AN IMPORTANT VITAMIN AND MINERAL SOURCE

Nutrients in Fruits. Among the nutrients to be found in fruits are potassium, magnesium, and traces of other minerals. There are large amounts of vitamin A in green and yellow fruits, and of course citrus fruits are rich sources of vitamin C. Other fruits high in vitamin C include papayas, strawberries, and guavas. The richest source of vitamin C, however, is acerola cherries, which are native to the West Indies. These cherries contain the highest vitamin-C concentration when they are green; when they ripen and turn red, they may look more tempting, but their vitamin-C content is lower. Acerola cherries have a pleasant, tart flavor that lends itself well to use in preserves and drinks. The juice is often mixed with other fruit juices, and is also used to make vitamin-C tablets.

Of course, fruits are also a source of natural sugar, satisfying a child's desire for something sweet without the dangers of refined sugar. Because they are eaten raw, fruits also provide bulk in the diet in the form of fiber, or cellulose, aiding in proper digestion and elimination.

FRESH FRUITS BEST

Fresh Versus Preserved Fruits. Thanks to our temperate climate and our vast transportation network, we are able to enjoy fresh fruits year round. These are generally vastly preferable to canned and frozen products. When fruit is prepared for commercial canning, it is dipped in lye to remove the skins. Moreover, the heat used in canning destroys some of the vitamins in fruit, and the cans themselves may leach tin and lead into the foods. Even though freezing doesn't destroy as many of the nutrients, fruit is often washed with detergent as a preparation for freezing and then dipped in a sulfur-dioxide solution to prevent brownish discoloration. This chemical, which is also used to preserve the color and flavor of dried fruit, can produce symptoms including nausea, headache, backache, and anemia in susceptible individuals.

FRUITS GASSED TO SIMULATE RIPENESS

Contaminants in Fresh Fruit. Although fresh fruit is certainly the best, we must be alert to the practices of some growers when we select our fruit at the market. The vitamin content of most fruit increases with its ripeness, and many of the fruits in the market have been picked before they are ripe. To lend the appearance of ripeness, many kinds of unripe fruits are sprayed with ethylene gas. You may have wondered how the fruit you buy in the market can be so flavorless when it looks so ripe; it's because it *is* unripe, the gassing process having imparted the artificial color of ripeness. Some fruits, such as papayas, will never develop their true flavor if they are picked before they are ripe.

CHEMICAL CONTAMINATION OF MUCH FRUIT

As if the practice of gassing unripe fruit weren't bad enough, other unnatural substances have already had the opportunity to contaminate the fruit long before picking. Fruit may be grown in soil that has been depleted through overuse and treated with large quantities of chemical fertilizers. Then the fruit trees may be sprayed with pesticides, which collect on the skins of the fruit. Once the fruit has been picked, it may be given a protective coating of mineral oil, which is known to interfere with the absorption of dietary calcium and phosphorus and some vitamins, robbing the body of these necessary nutrients. Suspect as a possible cause of cancer, mineral oil was banned as a coating for fruit in Germany way back in 1938, but it continues to be used in the United States.

Now that you know what substances may be lurking on the skins of that shiny fruit you bought in the market, you can understand why it is so important to wash it thoroughly before putting it in your child's lunch box!

Apple products with no daminozide are put out by Mott's, Tree Top, Red Cheek and Veryfine. Also BABY FOOD Producers.

But fruit may also be covered with wax, to make it appear shiny and to protect it from bruising, even though this wax is suspected to contain a cancer-causing substance. This dangerous material cannot be easily removed by washing, but it can be removed by soaking in detergent for three to five minutes and then scrubbing thoroughly. The only sure protection may be to peel fruit you suspect of being waxed, which means losing the vitamins and minerals close to the skin; and of course there are some fruits, like strawberries, that can't be peeled.

Another assault on the skins of fruits takes the form of various dyes. Oranges, for example, are picked green and unripe, washed in detergent, sometimes bleached, and then dyed with Red Dye #2, which has been shown in experiments to be changed into a carcinogenic substance in the bodies of laboratory animals to which it was fed. Because this dye may penetrate into the orange itself, peeling is not a sure protection against it. And of course orange peel itself is sometimes used in foods such as marmalade, or grated in pastries. Recognizing that such dyes are dangerous, some countries have banned the use of artificially colored oranges. The United States regulatory agencies, sympathetic with agribusiness interests, have lagged far behind in protecting the health of our children in this regard.

PERFECT-LOOKING FRUIT MAY NOT BE THE SAFEST

We could go on and on with a list of the artificial treatments given to fruits. The point is not to scare you out of your wits but rather to let you know that through discriminating shopping it is still possible to buy fruit that hasn't been chemically treated. There are still growers who are producing fruit grown in good soil, without the use of harmful pesticides, dyes, gases, and waxes. You may be able to find organically grown fruit in a health-food store. By all means don't shy away from fruit that is not uniform in size and that has little blemishes; very often this may mean that the fruit has been grown for its nutritional value and flavor rather than for uniform appearance. Look for fruits that are labeled "vine-ripened" or "tree ripened"; this means that they were not picked before they were ripe but rather allowed to develop their full flavor naturally on the plant. Buying fruit when it is in season is another way to be a little more sure that it hasn't been ripened by artificial means.

MOST RIPE FRUITS NEED REFRIGERATION

Storing fresh fruit. We must add a note on storing fresh fruit. Once fruit is ripe, its vitamin A, B$_2$, and C content will gradually deteriorate unless it is refrigerated. An exception is thick-skinned fruit such as citrus fruits and bananas; because their skins protect them, these fruits can be kept at room temperature without losing their nutritional value.

UNSULFURED DRIED FRUITS PREFERABLE

Dried fruits. A rich and nourishing snack, dried fruits contain some of the nutrients of their fresh counterparts in concentrated form. Whether dried naturally by the sun or artificially in ovens, dried fruits have been valued since antiquity for their high energy value, rich flavors, and ease of storage and transportation. Most dried fruit sold today has been treated with sulfur dioxide to enhance its color. Eating as little as six or seven ounces of sulfured dried fruits on a daily basis might be enough to produce unpleasant sulfur-dioxide-toxicity symptoms, such as nausea, dizziness, and headache. You can avoid sulfured dried fruits by reading the labels, which must state if sulfur has been used in the preserving process. Health-food stores often carry unsulfured dried fruits in bulk. Although these unsulfured apricots, peaches, and other fruits may not have the bright colors of the sulfured variety, their chewy texture and complex sweetness appeal to many a youthful palate, while not producing excessive foul-smelling bowel gas.

LUNCH

Dairy Products

SOME CHILDREN INTOLERANT OF COW'S MILK

Milk. As we have already seen, human milk is the perfect food for infants, and cow's milk or dairy products continue to supply important nutrients for growing children, especially calcium. Some children are not able to tolerate cow's milk, either because of a true allergy to it (cow's milk is probably the most common food allergen in the United States) or because of a lactase deficiency that makes it difficult to digest lactose, a sugar contained in milk. In the case of the true allergies, it is sometimes helpful to substitute goat's milk or soy milk, which are available in some health-food stores. For lactose intolerance (see Book III for detailed symptoms), it may help to give your child *natural* yogurt, kefir, or other fermented dairy products instead of whole milk.* These milk products, already partially digested through bacterial action, are low in lactose, and so may not upset your child's digestive system the same way that milk does. (A tip: naturally aged cheddar cheese contains very little lactose, and warm milk may not produce the symptoms of cramps and bloating seen with cold milk.)

How Much Milk Should a Child Drink Each Day? Getting the recommended allowance of calcium in the

---

* Caution: Much commercial yogurt contains added lactose; see discussion on pages 85–86.

diet is not easy with children who dislike milk. The RDAs for calcium for different age groups are:

	Age	RDA
Infants:	0–6 months	360 mg
	6 mo.–1 yr.	540 mg
Children:	1–3 years	800 mg
	4–6 years	800 mg
	7–10 years	800 mg
	11–14 years	1200 mg
	15–18 years	1200 mg
Adults:	19–50 years	800 mg

ALTERNATIVES TO MILK OUTLINED

To get this much calcium each day you may use the sample food plans outlined in Table 5, which follows.

CERTIFIED RAW MILK MOST NUTRITIOUS

How Is Milk Processed? The milk available in most markets today has been *pasteurized;* that is, it has been partially sterilized by heating it to destroy harmful bacteria. Unfortunately, in the process of this heating, vitamins A, C, E, and some B vitamins are partially destroyed or altered. In addition, beneficial bacteria are killed along with dangerous types. Some years ago, the U.S. Department of Agriculture reported that calves fed only on pasteurized cow's milk all died within three months on this diet. Even though our children have other sources of nutrients in their diets besides milk, it is always advisable to avoid foods that have been processed in such a way that they have lost some of their nutritional value. For this reason, you may want to look for raw milk in a reputable health-food store. The sale of raw milk is regulated by local ordinance in most states, and so it may not be available in your community. Some health officials

TABLE 5
Dietary Sources of Calcium*

DIET PLAN A		DIET PLAN B		DIET PLAN C		DIET PLAN D	
Food	**Calcium mg**	**Food**	**Calcium mg**	**Food**	**Calcium mg**	**Food**	**Calcium mg**
Milk or yogurt, 1½ pints	855	Milk or yogurt, 1 pint	570	Milk or yogurt, ½ pint	285	Cheddar cheese, 1½ oz.	337
		Cottage cheese, 2 tbsp.	52	Cheddar cheese, 1 oz.	225	Whole-wheat bread, 4 slices	92
		4 slices whole-wheat bread	92	Whole-wheat bread, 5 slices	95	1 medium egg	27
				Orange juice, 8 oz.	24	Baked beans with molasses, ½ cup	82
		1 medium orange	62	Broccoli, ⅔ cup	88	4 apricots, dried	40
		¾ cup green beans, cooked	45	2 large figs, dried	50	Salmon, red, canned, with bones, ⅖ cup	259
			821	Peanut butter, 2 tbsp.	22		837
				3–4 pitted dates (1 oz.)	22		
					811		

*Adapted from Briggs and Calloway (1979).

claim that raw milk is a common source of salmonella infections, and for this reason you should use only *certified* raw milk, which an independent assayer has stated to be free of pathogens.

Homogenized milk is produced by breaking up and evenly distributing the globules of fat and the shreds of casein (a milk protein) in the milk to achieve a uniform texture, which supposedly makes the milk easier to digest. Unfortunately there is a suspicion that these smaller fat globules lodge in arterial walls. For this reason, again we recommend raw, unhomogenized milk and dairy foods. Obviously, raw milk from unknown or questionable sources is to be avoided.

CHILDREN NEED FAT IN MILK

Skim milk has a lower fat content than whole milk, some of the fat having been removed before pasteurization. With the reduction of fat content, however, important fat-soluble vitamins, including A, D, E, and K, are also removed. Children need the valuable nutrients carried in butterfat, and so there is very little reason to give your child milk containing reduced quantities of fat. Also, for proper calcium absorption, some fat is necessary. Some children, however, have difficulty digesting the fat in milk, and skim milk may be a solution for them.

Low-fat milk contains even less fat, between 0.5 percent and 2 percent as compared with 3–6 percent for whole cow's milk. Low-fat milk is low in cholesterol, which is not a relevant consideration for children except those with certain familial predispositions to atherosclerotic disease. In any event, low-fat milk should not be given to children without good medical reason.

SOME BUTTER DYED YELLOW

Butter. Nothing can replace the rich, creamy butter that is made from farm-fresh cream. With the food industry's customary chemical ingenuity, butter producers have learned that chemical additives can be used to "salvage" stale, soured cream, and, with the addition of other chemicals to disguise bad odors and the signs of bacterial action, to make a product that is still sold as butter. The desirable yellow color of fresh butter, which comes from the cows' diet of grass, is sometimes achieved artificially through the use of coal-tar dyes, and salt may be added to slow the growth of yeast and molds. You don't need to settle for this poor approximation of the real thing, and to ensure that you are buying wholesome butter made from fresh cream, look for the label "fresh creamery butter" on the packages in your market's dairy case. Reject any butter or cheese that is labeled "artificially colored."

Even less acceptable is *margarine*. Although it may be lower in price than butter, there is no justification for giving this synthetic mixture of potentially harmful ingredients to your child. We shall discuss the process by which margarine is made in the "Dinner" section below.

FERMENTED MILK PRODUCTS DESCRIBED

Other Milk Products. *Buttermilk* was traditionally a product derived from heavy cream, consisting of the liquid that was left behind after the butter had been churned out. The product sold as buttermilk today is the result of modern processing techniques through which skim or pasteurized milk is fermented and then churned together with butter. The only reason this product is preferred is for taste (bitter, due to lactic acid), and for those unable to digest unfermented milk products.

Many children enjoy the tangy, slightly acidic flavor of *yogurt,* which contains all the nutrients present in milk but in partly broken down and more readily digestible form. Yogurt is produced by inoculating milk with a bacterial culture that multiplies to form yogurt. Yogurt is believed by many people to promote health by encouraging the growth of valuable bacteria in the intestine.

Yogurt may be made from low-fat or whole milk; for the same reasons we discussed with milk itself (better calcium absorption and more vitamins), the whole-milk variety is preferable for your child. A dietary staple in India and the Middle East, yogurt is a perfect complement for the spicy foods of those cultures. You can serve it plain, or combined with fruit, vegetables, or even meat dishes. Beware of the fruit-flavored yogurts in your supermarket. The fruit they contain is, of course, highly processed and of little nutritional value; but even worse, these yogurts generally contain much sugar as well. Why substitute the excessive, syrupy sweetness of refined sugar for the natural sweetness of fresh, ripe fruit? Artificial colors also abound in "flavored" yogurts.

You (and perhaps your child) might want to try making yogurt at home. Many cookbooks contain instructions for producing this healthful product, and kits are now widely available to make the process as convenient as possible. It's a fascinating experience for children to be able to watch "live food" being produced right in their own kitchen!

Kefir is another fermented milk product, with somewhat the same tangy taste as yogurt. Again, watch out for kefir products containing added sweeteners and artificial ingredients.

PROCESSED CHEESES CONTAIN MUCH WATER

Cheese. Cheese-making is an old art, involving the combination of acid-forming bacteria and milk-curdling enzymes with pure milk. Modern processed cheeses are far inferior to these natural, healthful traditional products. Although there is really very little reason to buy any of them, an understanding of the names applied to processed cheeses will help you to find your way through the confusing maze of cheese products in your supermarket. The differences in the names—"processed cheese," "cheese food," "cheese spread," "imitation cheese spread," "cheese product"—reflect the quantity of water that is contained in the cheese. Obviously, the more water, the less nutritional value the product contains. According to government standards, for example, American cheese is allowed to have 43 percent water content and must have 27 percent butterfat; "cheese food" has more water and less butterfat, and "cheese spreads" may contain as little as 20 percent butterfat.

DRUGGED COWS PRODUCE DRUGGED MILK

Contaminants in milk and milk products. At the risk of sounding like chronic alarmists, we must point out that dairy products are not exempt from the tampering that seems to be a universal theme in the food industry today. The questionable practice of pasteurization may remove some of the bacteria in milk, but food technology has stepped in with some other potentially harmful substances to make up for it. Dairy cows are susceptible to mastitis, or inflammation of the breast tissue, which may decrease milk production, and so dairy farmers treat their herds with penicillin. This antibiotic passes through the cow's body and into its milk, and for some people it can have very serious health effects. Some individuals who are allergic to penicillin may develop severe reactions to milk containing this antibiotic. It is now accepted wisdom among the medical profession that penicillin should only be used in case of infection, and should never be given on a regular basis, as may happen through the daily use of penicillin-contaminated milk. Not only does such constant ingestion of penicillin increase one's susceptibility to infection by penicillin-resistant organisms, but beneficial bacteria in the intestines may also be killed. To increase the cows' milk output, they may also be given hormones such as oestrin, and they may receive tranquilizers to relax them and increase their yield. Cows may graze on grasses sprayed with DDT and other pesticides. All these substances make their way into the milk we drink. Even the detergent used to wash milking equipment can end up in the carton in the dairy case.

Beyond the nutritional objections to pasteurization, it is obvious that *certified* raw milk, produced by inspected dairies, may be the only alternative to the contaminated versions of this very necessary dietary item. Your favorite health-food store may be able to advise you where to obtain milk that is free from chemical and pharmaceutical tampering.

ICE CREAM AN INFREQUENT TREAT

Ice cream. When it's made from the traditional high-quality combination of ingredients including milk, cream, eggs, and fresh fruits, ice cream can be a nutritious and satisfying food. When properly made, ice cream will provide your child with protein, calcium, phosphorus, and vitamins. Of course, it also contains sugar as a sweetener, although a number of smaller ice-cream manufacturers are now making their products with honey in place of sugar. In any case, because it is a sweet, ice cream should not be eaten more frequently than once weekly. (For a nondairy, sugarless alternative to ice cream try the recipe for chocolate ice cream in the "Sweet Things" section of Book IV.)

AIR AND CHEMICALS CALLED ICE CREAM

As with cheeses, there are many imitations of ice cream on the market that are only the most distant relatives of this healthful food. Ice cream and related products are for some reason excluded from federal labeling regulations, the only ingredients needing to be listed being flavors. However, FDA standards do define what ingredients may be used in ice cream or frozen desserts, specifying the minimum amount of butterfat and the maximum amount of air these products may contain. You may be surprised to discover that inexpensive ice cream contains about 50 percent air, in the form of gelatins and gums added to the mixture! The same FDA standards also allow all sorts of very non-ice-creamy ingredients to be used in specified amounts, including seaweed products, plant gums, and chemical additives of dubious safety and no nutritional value. Such products are a far cry from the good, old-fashioned, hand-cranked ice cream of the past. The best thing to do when you shop for ice cream is to be prepared to pay a little bit more and to study the labels carefully, selecting only the brands that state that all ingredients are natural and that don't use stabilizers, emulsifiers, colorings, or artificial flavors.

Other so-called ice-cream products get even farther away from real ice cream. "Milkshakes," for example, are a mixture of milk and ice cream, but they may contain ice milk, which may be little more than a mixture of artificial ingredients. Stick to the real thing here. It may be cheaper in the long run.

Sandwiches

We've already covered some of the main ingredients of your child's lunchtime sandwich, which must always start with nutritious, stone-ground whole-grain bread. From our discussion of cheeses, you know which products to avoid, and in the section on breakfast meats you were warned about the dangers of nitrites and nitrates in such processed luncheon meats as bologna, salami, and ham. Other meats that might be used in sandwiches are discussed in the "Dinner" section. Egg salad is another popular and nutritious sandwich filling. As we'll see later, sprouts make a crunchy and healthful addition to many sandwiches.

Now let's take a look at the components of one of the big favorites with children, the peanut-butter-and-jelly sandwich.

REAL PEANUT BUTTER BELONGS IN REFRIGERATOR

Peanut Butter. Real peanut butter, made from ground-up peanuts, with perhaps a little added peanut oil or salt, is a nutritious food. It supplies good, though not complete, protein, as well as unsaturated fatty acids and vitamins. Such peanut butter, incidentally, must be kept refrigerated to prevent its valuable oils from becoming rancid. Don't sacrifice the nutritional value of good peanut butter for greater ease of spreading by keeping it at room temperature.

COMMERCIAL PEANUT BUTTERS EXAMINED

Unfortunately, the peanut butter in your supermarket is generally quite different from the wholesome products we have just described. Instead of containing healthful unsaturated oils, these commercial peanut butters are usually hydrogenated into saturated fats. (We shall see later why hydrogenation of oils constitutes a threat to our children's health.) Often the oil used in commercial peanut butters is cottonseed oil, which has a higher than average danger of containing pesticides since cotton (a fiber plant, not a food plant!) is usually sprayed to protect against weevils. These inferior products may also contain sugar, and to prevent the separation of the oil they may also contain emulsifiers, which can lead to irritation of the digestive system and other problems. In addition to these chemical manipulations, you may be surprised to learn that commercial peanut butters are allowed by law to contain rather alarming levels of insect fragments and rodent hairs!

If your market doesn't carry genuine peanut butter, containing nothing but peanuts and perhaps a little oil, you might want to look in a health-food store for peanut butter sold in bulk, preferably freshly made. Another alternative is to invest in a peanut grinder and make it yourself at home. This will provide yet another opportunity for your child to participate in the fun and learning experience of helping to make wholesome, genuine food rather than thinking it all originates in jars and cans.

OTHER NUT BUTTERS OFFER VARIETY

While you're in the health-food store, incidentally, you might take a look at some of the other nut and seed "butters" they have for sale. Though more expensive than peanut butter, such products as cashew butter and tahini (made from sesame seeds) make for an interesting change of pace. In the "Dressings and Spreads" section of Book IV we provide a simple recipe for nut or seed butter, which can be made in a blender, as well as instructions for making some high-protein bean spreads.

SUGARLESS JAMS CAN BE MADE

Jams, Jellies, Fruit Butters, and Preserves. There is no denying that peanut butter goes well with jam or jelly. These fruit preserves are usually made by boiling fresh fruit with large quantities of sugar, sometimes with the addition of pectin as a thickening agent to supplement the natural pectin in the fruit. Here is another area where you might want to explore making nutritious foods at home rather than relying on the overly sugared commercial products. Most fruit preserves rely on sugar to help the thickening process, but you can make jellies, jams, preserves, and fruit butters without sugar, relying on the natural sweetness of the fruit. See our recipes in Book IV under "Dressings and Spreads" for a good start in learning to make sugarless jams and fruit butters.

Eliminating Junk Food from the Lunchbox

JUNK FOOD'S APPEAL CREATED BY ADVERTISING

As we saw in the case of the Castlemont School, some schools have become so concerned about the nutritional dangers of sweet, gooey, prepackaged cakes, cookies, and other baked goods, and products like potato and corn chips, that they don't allow them to be sold on campus. We'll see later on in our discussion of potato chips and similar greasy snacks that they contain a multiplicity of questionable ingredients and are produced under less than healthful conditions. As we move now to a consideration of sweets in general, we will see that there *are* healthful alternatives to the junk food that is a combination of high refined-sugar content, artificial flavorings and colorings, and other valueless ingredients and dangerous chemicals often promoted directly to children. As we shall see, wholesome cookies, pastries, and other baked goods, made from fresh, natural ingredients, and other nonsugared sweets are available, easy to prepare, and part of our preventive diet. Remember, if it does not taste good, your youngsters will not eat it, no matter how "good" it is supposed to be.

AFTER-SCHOOL REFUELING

*Pleasant words are as a honeycomb, sweet
to the soul, and health to the bones.*
PROVERBS 16:24

AFTERNOON SNACK SUGGESTIONS GIVEN

It's snack time once again when your child arrives home from school in the afternoon. There are available to you many wholesome, nutritious choices offering a wide range of flavors, textures, and caloric content. Some possibilities include raw vegetables, fresh fruits, raisins and other dried fruits, cheese, unsalted popcorn, small sandwiches, natural ice cream, raw unsalted nuts and seeds, whole-grain and graham crackers (without preservatives), home-baked cakes, cookies and pretzels, no-sugar granola, trail mix, and of course fruit juice and milk. With such a wide range of appealing choices, there's little excuse for resorting to junk food that will only destroy your child's appetite for a well-rounded dinner.

But why do we object so vehemently to sugary treats? Let's examine in a little more detail the case that is building against refined sugar.

Sweets

INSECTS AND FRUITS PRODUCED EARLY SWEETENERS

Sweeteners have been eaten since prehistoric times. An important element of the diet, natural sugars provide energy in the form of calories to support body function. Sugars also make it possible for us to enjoy some foods that would otherwise be too bitter or too tart. Until fairly recently, however, the sweeteners used by man were the natural, unrefined sugars derived from fruits, plants, and honey, and the quantity consumed was far lower than what is used in the United States today.

Honey was the most common sweetener used prior to the introduction of refined sugars, while the carob (in Egypt), dates, figs, grapes, and other sweet fruits were popular sugar substitutes. Manna, the Biblical "bread of life" to the ancient Israelites, was actually a sweet secretion of an insect, which collected on the twigs of the tamarisk tree. The Bedouins still gather this naturally sweet food and make a puree from it.

MODERN MAN ADDICTED TO SUGAR

Yes, sweets have been with us for a long time, but never before in history have people eaten as much as we do in the Western nations: about 120 pounds of refined sweeteners yearly, or nearly 25 percent of our total caloric intake! This is 30 times more than the average American colonist ate in 1700. How did we develop such a craving?

SUGAR-REFINING ELIMINATES NUTRIENTS

Sugars are formed in plants through the process of photosynthesis, and some plants, such as sugar cane, sugar beets, and the maple store large quantities of sugar that can then be utilized by man. The refined white sugar we eat today is known as sucrose, and is derived from sugar cane and sugar beets. In its raw, unrefined form, the sugar in cane is a nourishing food, containing fiber, B vitamins, iron, calcium, and other minerals. Many primitive people regularly consume sugar cane as an important part of their diet. (Sugar cane is an interesting table item, worth buying if only for the discussions it can stimulate. Children love to know what things really are, and this natural product, the source of all cane sugar, is a good lesson in nutritional realism.)

In the refining process, the sweet sap from sugar cane is subjected to chemical treatment, boiling, and crystallization to produce dark-brown raw sugar, leaving behind a sticky residue known as molasses, which is rich in nutrients. The dark, raw sugar, which is still quite nutritious, is then refined into white sugar through a series of harsh processes that strip it of its protein, vitamins, minerals, fiber, and organic acids and leave a white crystalline substance containing little but "empty calories"— meaning that there is little or nothing of nutritional value to accompany this caloric energy. Table 6 compares the nutrients in white sugar, molasses, honey, and maple sugar; the numbers eloquently demonstrate how empty the calories of white sugar really are.

TABLE 6
Nutrient Content of Sugars and Other Sweeteners*
(Composition per 100 g or 3½ oz.)

	White Sugar (Granulated)	(Beet or Cane)	Molasses (Third Extraction or Blackstrap)	Honey (Strained or Extracted)	Maple Sugar
Minerals:	mg	mg	mg	mg	mg
Calcium	0	85	684	5	143
Phosphorus	0	19	84	6	11
Iron	0.1	3.4	16.1	0.5	1.4
Sodium	1.0	30	96	5	14
Potassium	3.0	344	2927	51	242
Vitamins:					
Thiamine	0	0.01	0.11	trace	—
Riboflavin	0	0.03	0.19	0.04	—
Niacin	0	0.2	2.0	0.3	—

*Source: "Composition of Foods," Agriculture Handbook No. 8, U.S. Dept. of Agriculture. Values given vary in other sources.

EXCESSIVE SUGAR PROMOTES MALNUTRITION

What are the dangers in consuming these empty calories? The highly refined sugar we eat today can become a substitute for the more complete foods that contain the essential nutrients such as proteins and vitamins that our bodies require. Our bodies can convert the food we eat into glucose, the form of sugar that circulates in the blood and supplies energy to our cells, but we are not able to manufacture protein from sugar. We must ingest enough protein in our foods to ensure an adequate supply of essential amino acids as building blocks for our cells and tissues, and foods such as refined sugar, which contain no nutrients, may discourage the intake of adequate protein that is of particular importance in a rapidly growing child.

Advertisers are always telling us that the sugar in candies and other sweets provides "quick energy," but this energy is of little value in itself if it isn't supplemented by a balanced diet. The fact remains that the more sugar we eat, the less likely we are to get the essential nutrients in our diets since we feel satisfied by the sweets and don't eat the basic foods.

SUGAR A CULPRIT IN MODERN SCOURGES

Besides its adverse influence on dietary patterns, high sugar intake has been directly implicated in a number of serious diseases, including coronary-artery disease, diabetes, appendicitis, and cancer of the digestive tract. The role of excess sugar in obesity is well known. There is evidence, also, that sugar in any form (not just refined sugar) may produce hyperactivity in some susceptible individuals. Of course, sugar is also the number-one villain in tooth decay.

HIDDEN SUGAR IN PROCESSED FOODS

You may object to the above argument, saying that surely your family isn't spooning a third of a pound of sugar apiece out of the bowl each day (120 pounds yearly). But remember that 70 percent of this amount is in the form of refined sweeteners added by manufacturers to processed foods and beverages. The only way you can really be sure you're eliminating or reducing the refined sugar in your family's diet is to stick with fresh fruits, vegetables, meats, poultry, and fish, keeping packaged foods to a minimum. Once you've been alerted to the presence of sugar, "corn sweeteners," "natural sweeteners," and such in processed foods, you can develop a regular habit of reading the labels. You'll be amazed to discover there's sugar not only in such obviously sweet products as pastries, candies, desserts, and cookies but also in many "natural" breakfast cereals, crackers, breads, baking mixes, soups, cured meats, salad dressings, ketchup, and canned and frozen fruits and vegetables— to name only a few. Remember that the ingredient that is listed first on the label is the one that's present in the greatest quantity. As we've seen, some breakfast cereals contain more sugar than any other ingredient. Even in the field of health products, you'll find sugar coating on vitamin pills and on prescription drugs!

BROWN SUGAR NO BETTER THAN WHITE

Brown sugar. Some people think that brown sugar is more nutritious than white sugar, taking its brown color as a sign that it's more "natural," and similar to raw sugar. This impression is further fostered by some food manufacturers who proudly proclaim that they use brown sugar in their products. Actually brown sugar is for all practical purposes nothing but empty calories, just like white sugar. The process for making brown sugar begins with the boiled sugar syrup; instead of being crystallized to form white sugar, it is mixed with a little molasses and then filtered and boiled in a vacuum, yielding brown crystals that are 96 percent sucrose. As water evaporates, the syrup becomes darker and darker, and it is crystallized to form sugars of various colors depending on how concentrated it is. Obviously, nothing in this process has added much to the nutritional value of the devitalized sugar syrup.

So-called "raw," "yellow-D," or "turbinado" sugar is also little more than 96 percent sucrose. Like brown sugar, these varieties are white sugar with a small amount of added molasses.

GLUCOSE ADDED TO COMMON FOODS

Glucose. Refined sugar, as we have seen, is sucrose. Glucose, also known as dextrose, is another form of sugar, which is found in corn syrup. Because it is absorbed into the bloodstream much more rapidly than other sugars, glucose is used for intravenous feeding of hospital patients. Glucose is much less sweet than sucrose, and so it is possible to eat large quantities of this sugar without being aware of its presence in your food. Glucose, or dextrose, is added to many packaged and canned foods, including canned fruits and juices, preserves, cheeses, condensed milk, ketchup, and dried fruits, as well as the more obvious sweets.

FRUCTOSE OFFERS MINIMAL ADVANTAGES OVER SUCROSE

Fructose. As a reaction against the known dangers of excessive sucrose in the diet, many health-food stores are now selling fructose, a sugar found in honey and many fruits. Fructose *is* a bit easier on the system than sucrose. While sucrose requires the secretion of insulin to be metabolized, fructose can be metabolized and absorbed without insulin. A word of caution, though: *diabetics beware!* You must take insulin to metabolize fructose, just as you do with sucrose. So avoid all refined sugars.

Nondiabetics might also profitably avoid fructose, which is increasingly found in yogurt and "health food" soft drinks. It is still a refined sugar, albeit easier on our system than others, but it is devoid of fiber and other nutrients found in the unrefined carbohydrates. Besides, you can't chew fructose, and chewing is good for our teeth, not to mention our nervous system.

REAL MAPLE SYRUP A VANISHING FOOD

Maple and Other Pancake Syrups. The maple tree is one of the less common sources of sugar, and maple sugar in the form of syrup is a traditional accompaniment for pancakes and waffles. However, the syrup we're using on our pancakes today is likely to contain only negligible amounts of real maple syrup, and if you look at the labels on pancake syrups, you'll find that they're really nothing but mixtures of chemicals. Some syrups contain no maple syrup at all and are merely combinations of artificial flavoring with corn and sugar syrups. Even 100-percent-pure maple syrup is of limited nutritional value, since the long heating process to which the sap is subjected destroys most of its nutrients. For those who like maple syrup, it's a good idea to look for 100-percent-pure syrup that is labeled "untreated." American maple-syrup producers often put poisonous formaldehyde pellets in the tapholes to kill insects in their maple trees. This practice is illegal in Canada, and is avoided by some producers of maple syrup in Vermont; so to be sure you're avoiding this dangerous chemical, you might want to buy Canadian maple syrup, or perhaps Vermont syrup that specifically states that this practice has been avoided.

HONEY NUTRIENT-RICH

Honey. A good substitute for refined sugar is honey, which unlike most other sweetening agents retains most of its minerals, vitamins, and other nutrients in its pure state. It's unlikely to contain pesticides, since honeybees are very susceptible to pesticides and will usually die before they get back to the hive if they have come into contact with these chemicals. The natural sweetness of honey protects it against the growth of molds, and so it doesn't require added preservatives. Table 6, on page 95, will allow you to compare the nutrient value of honey with that of other sweeteners.

SOME HONEYS TOXIC

Even a pure food like honey, under unfavorable conditions, can be dangerous. The nectar of certain plants, including the mountain laurel, azalea, yellow jasmine, and some rhododendrons, results in honey that can be toxic to humans. Such toxic honeys have been responsible for poisonings since ancient times, but we are largely protected against this danger by the fact that the bees themselves are often killed by these toxic honeys, and that commercial beekeepers are careful to eliminate any plants that may produce toxic honeys from the neighborhood of their hives.

UNHEATED HONEY ADVISED FOR ALL BUT INFANTS

Honey has to ripen in the comb to develop its full flavor. To hasten this ripening process, some producers heat the honey, but since heating destroys vitamins and other nutrients, it's wise to buy unprocessed, raw, unfiltered and unheated honey. Such honey may be slightly cloudy and may have a tendency to crystallize, but it's greatly preferable to the clear, fluid honeys that generally have less flavor and are less nutritious. There is an important exception to this general rule, however. Raw, unheated honey may present an inherent danger to infants, whose digestive systems are unable to destroy potentially harmful bacteria that may be present in large numbers in raw honey. While older children are perfectly capable of consuming this natural sweet without harm, raw honey has been implicated in the deaths of infants, and so *only cooked honey should be given to infants.*

CHEWING GUM A PETROLEUM PRODUCT

Candies and Other Sweets. We must be constantly on the alert against the relentless marketing strategies of the people who are pushing sugar products. Storekeepers are instructed to have sweets at strategic locations throughout their markets where they will be at eye level for children and will be bought as impulse items. And it's not just the obviously harmful candy bars that should be avoided; give a second thought, too, to what goes into chewing gum before buying it for your child. Originally, chewing-gum base was made from materials derived from natural plant sources, such as chicle. Today, the gum base used in chewing gums may include a number of petroleum derivatives suspected of causing cancer. Additional petroleum products may be added as softeners, and the gum may also contain the antioxidants BHA and BHT, as well as artificial flavors and colors. The sugar content of chewing gum, close to 60 percent, is a further reason for avoiding these products.

NATURAL SWEETS APPEAL TO YOUTHFUL PALATES

This is not to say that all sweets and candies are necessarily harmful. Candies such as those sold in health-food stores may be made from natural ingredients such as nuts, raisins, coconut, dates, peanut butter, carob, oats, and wheat germ, and sweetened with honey. Such sweets can have real, concentrated nutritional value. Even in health-food stores, however, be sure to read the labels and be sure to avoid refined sugars or other harmful ingredients.

Of course, even natural sweets such as honey should be eaten only in moderation; *any* sweetener will contribute to harmful eating habits in your child if used in excess. It may surprise you to learn that sweets can be made entirely without added sweeteners of any kind. The recipes in the "Sweet Things" section of Book IV will guide you in making many safe and healthful treats at home, using only the natural sweetness of fruit.

SACCHARIN WIDELY USED THOUGH SUSPECT

Artificial Sweeteners. Perhaps, as an alternative to refined sugar in your child's diet, you might be tempted to turn to artificial sweeteners such as saccharin for certain purposes, as in soft drinks, canned fruits, and "sugarless" gums. These products, however, must be viewed with extreme suspicion in light of the present experimental evidence against them. The two most widely used artificial sweeteners in this country are saccharin, which is 300 times sweeter than sugar by weight, and cyclamates, which are 30 times sweeter than sugar. In 1969, after a great deal of controversy and debate, the use of cyclamates was severely restricted by the FDA, so that these artificial sweeteners are now classified as drugs and have been removed from the list of food additives "Generally Regarded as Safe." Although the food industry persisted in protesting that cyclamates were harmless, researchers found that these chemicals produced a wide range of adverse effects in laboratory animals, including slowed growth rates, stillbirths, laxative effects, liver damage, and interference with certain medicines.

Saccharin, a coal-tar derivative, remains on the market in spite of evidence that it causes cancer of the bladder in experimental animals. Its use has been forbidden in foods in France and Germany for nearly a century, and other countries have banned it more recently. Today saccharin is the sweetener used in diet drinks and dietetic foods in the United States, and because of its highly suspect status, these foods should not be a part of the diet of a growing child.

RECIPES PROVIDED FOR HEALTHFUL BAKED GOODS

Pastries, Cookies, and Cakes. What more worthless combination can you imagine than the empty calories of refined sugar and of starchy white flour, all mixed together with artificial flavors and colors, preservatives, and hydrogenated oils? Such are the concoctions that tempt our youngsters on the junk-food racks of the corner candy store and the supermarket. Yet even those home baked cakes, pies, and cookies so lovingly prepared according to Grandmother's favorite recipe are often guilty of excessive reliance on refined and processed ingredients that have been stripped of their nutritional value. As creative cooks become more aware of the devitalization of our staple foods, there is a growing interest in developing recipes for nutritious cakes, cookies, pies, and other baked goods using honey or fruit in place of refined sugar, and whole-wheat flour and other nutritious whole-grain products in place of white flour. A good way to start learning to bake without refined sugar, white flour, and fats is to use the "Sweet Things" recipes in Book IV. As the table of ingredient exchanges indicates, the quantities of ingredients will sometimes require some adjustment, as may the baking time, if you substitute ingredients in your own recipes. The texture of the resultant baked goods may also be a little different from the original, but the recipes for sweets from the Weimar Kitchen in Book IV have all the flavor and aroma, plus the chewiness, that children love. You will find these recipes foolproof for creating wholesome, satisfying, delicious sweets for that occasional treat at a meal or at snack time, for your children and yourself!

Nuts and Seeds

Raw, unsalted nuts and seeds are an excellent snack for children, high in protein and rich in unsaturated fatty acids and B vitamins. Vastly preferable to candies, these wholesome foods won't inhibit the appetite or produce dental cavities.

HOW TO AVOID RANCID NUTS

Because they contain essential oils, nuts become rancid if kept for a long time, leading to the destruction of their vitamins A, C, E, and some B vitamins. Avoid the packets of roasted and salted nuts available at candy counters, since the chances of rancidity are increased even further by the fact that they were usually cooked in oil. Similarly, heated nut dispensers often serve to mask the fact that nuts are rancid and stale. Of course, it's a good idea to avoid all that added salt on these processed nuts as well.

It's much wiser to buy nuts unsalted in vacuum-packed cans, or in the shell. Since the food industry uses chemical treatments on some nuts in the shell to enhance their appearance, don't hesitate to buy the less-uniform, darker-looking walnuts and other nuts that are available at health-food stores; and by all means avoid the red-dyed pistachios.

Health-food stores also sell nuts in bulk out of their shells, as well as unroasted and unsalted pumpkin, sunflower, sesame, and other seeds. Trail mixes combine these ingredients with bits of dried fruit to produce a tasty, high-energy, high-nutrition snack.

DINNER

Better is a dinner of herbs where love is,
than a stalled ox and hatred therewith.

PROVERBS 14:30

Meat, Poultry, and Fish

CHILDREN'S PROTEIN SUPPLY MUST BE ASSURED

As we saw in Book I, adequate protein intake is absolutely essential to proper growth. About 20 percent of your child's calories should be in the form of protein. Table 7 lists common sources of protein, grouped according to their protein content, beginning with the lower-protein foods.

FLESHY FOODS OUR PRINCIPAL PROTEIN SOURCE

The most common sources of protein in your child's diet are probably meat, poultry, and fish. The complete proteins contained in these foods are broken down in the small intestine into their component amino acids, which then enter the bloodstream and are distributed throughout the body, where they are recombined into the substances needed for constructing and repairing the body's cells and tissues. Besides supplying these essential amino acids, which the body is not able to manufacture for itself, meats, fish, and poultry also contain calcium, iron, vitamin A, and the B vitamins thiamine, riboflavin, and niacin.

CHOLESTEROL NOT A DANGER FOR MOST CHILDREN

Fats and cholesterol. Meat is also a source of cholesterol, as well as of saturated fats, which when eaten in ex-

TABLE 7
Protein Content of Common Foods*
(Grouped according to percentage
of protein content)

5%	10%	15%
Beef juice	Brain	Sweetbread
Liver juice	Bacon	Lung
Oysters	Evaporated milk	Kidney
Whole milk	Bread	Flounder
Peas, fresh	Breakfast cereals	Pork
Lima beans, fresh		Egg
Apricots		Chocolate
		Oatmeal
		Macaroni

20%	25%	30%
Liver	Beef	Beef, dry
Tongue	Swiss cheese	American cheese
Fish	Lentils	Peanut butter
Chicken	Peanuts	
Turkey	Peas, dry	100%
Lamb		Gelatin, dry
Cottage cheese		
Cocoa		
Walnuts		
Lima beans, dry		

* After Kugelmass (1940).

cessive quantities can cause the liver to produce more cholesterol. This complex chemical is necessary for many important bodily functions. It is only when excess amounts of cholesterol are consumed in the food, with accompanying excess levels of cholesterol in the blood, that the risk of atherosclerotic heart disease is increased. We have already noted that egg yolks and butterfat are other important foods that are high in cholesterol. For most children there is no need for concern about eating reasonable quantities of these nutritious foods; however, we should repeat our earlier caution that special dietary restrictions may be appropriate in families with strong histories of hyperlipidemia.

LEAN MEATS BEST FOR ALL

Unfortunately, we in the United States have come to favor a kind of meat that is extremely high in fat content. The highest grade of meat in markets in this country is "prime," with other grades in descending order being "choice," "good," "standard," and "commercial." The main characteristic distinguishing one grade of meat from another is its fat content, with prime having the most "marbelization," or fat distributed throughout the meat! This means a higher content of saturated fats and cholesterol, and a relatively smaller proportion of the valuable protein for which meat is eaten. Even though there are no dangers inherent in your child's consuming reasonable amounts of saturated fats and cholesterol, there is certainly no reason to eat these nutrients in excess, and the best value for your food dollar will be obtained in the form of lean meats, well cooked to remove fat.

Contaminants in Meats. Many of the animals we eat are capable of carrying diseases that are a potential threat to humans. Pork, for example, can be a source of trichinosis and hog cholera, while salmonella and staphylococcus bacteria can be found in fresh and processed meats. Most disease-producing bacteria are destroyed by heat, and so all meats should always be thoroughly cooked.

MEAT NO LONGER EATEN FRESH-KILLED

In earlier times meat, fish, and poultry were generally eaten freshly caught or slaughtered; when they had to be stored, they would be preserved by drying, salting, or smoking. Today, with the centralized production of almost all the food we consume, meats need to be stored for longer periods and transported over greater distances, calling for new ways of preserving them. We have already seen that modern food technology has developed the use of nitrites and nitrates for such purposes, as well as other chemicals for concealing signs of decay and disease. The U.S. Department of Agriculture's program for inspecting meats looks for obvious defects such as bruises, fecal contamination, enlarged livers, and obvious signs of bacterial contamination, but the chemical contaminants in meats do not disturb government inspectors, and these present a real and hidden danger.

More than half the antibiotics sold in this country are used in animal feed for the suppression of bacterial reproduction so that animals grow faster. Just as the penicillin fed to dairy cows ends up in their milk, so do the antibiotics fed to meat-producing animals end up in their meat. You are already familiar with the dangers such antibiotics can present to people who are sensitive to them, and how they can disturb the balance of beneficial and harmful bacteria in our bodies.

DANGEROUS HORMONE CONTAMINATES AMERICAN BEEF

Another cause for serious concern is the meat producers' practice of adding the female sex hormone diethylstilbestrol, or DES, to the feed of cattle and poultry. Used to produce a rapid fatty-weight gain in these animals prior to slaughter, DES has been shown to induce tumors, and to stop the growth of children. This hormone has been banned in many countries; in fact, Canada has refused to import American beef, mutton, and lamb because we allow DES to be added to the animals' feed. In response, our cattle industry has decided to produce DES-free meat, but only for export to Canada, while we in the United States must continue to buy DES-contaminated meat!

SUPERVISING GRINDING OF MEATS ADVISED

What's in That Hamburger? A favorite meat of children, hamburger can present some additional problems beyond those that may already exist in the meat from which it is made. The grinding of meat breaks down the tissues, and the fluid that escapes from the cells provides an excellent breeding ground for bacteria. Fortunately, cooking will destroy most bacteria in hamburger, but you must be careful to cook this meat well. Hamburger also often contains large quantities of fat, and butchers sometimes color low-grade ground beef with beef blood to conceal its high fat content. When you buy a hamburger in a restaurant, there's very little way of knowing what it contains, but when you buy ground beef to cook at home, your best protection is to select a lean piece of chuck or round steak and watch the butcher grind it in front of you. The ideal solution, of course, is to have a meat grinder at home and make your own fresh-ground hamburger from low-fat cuts of quality meat.

SOME HOT DOGS SAFE

Hot Dogs. Another food that is very popular with children, hot dogs require even more critical caution than hamburger. Usually made from some of the worst scraps from the slaughterhouse, they may also contain dangerous nitrites as well as other chemical additives and nonmeat "fillers." The designation "kosher" on hot dogs is no longer an assurance of food quality (these also contain dangerous preservatives). The only choice is to pay *more* for nitrite-free hot dogs, which are increasingly available. These are usually preserved with vitamin C, an added bonus.

CHICKENS FED ARSENIC

Poultry. Chicken, turkey, duck, and other poultry are a potential source of nutritious protein, often with lower fat content than red meats (assuming the skin is discarded); but, as with red meats, there is still a danger that we are ingesting harmful substances with our protein. Although an inspection program for poultry was established in 1968, the emphasis of these inspections is more on appearance than on hidden contamination by bacteria and dangerous chemicals, which means that even a good grade of poultry is not necessarily free of these dangers. Ninety percent of all commercially raised chickens are given feed that contains arsenic, which stimulates growth and egg production and makes the skin a more desirable yellow color. Traces of this poison end up in the chicken we eat, especially in the liver, since that organ removes the arsenic from the system. Arsenic has been established as a cancer-causing agent in man, and so there is real danger if we eat large amounts of poultry contaminated with this substance. By all means drop chopped chicken livers from your recipes, no matter how delicious.

CAREFUL SHOPPING FOR POULTRY ADVISED

The feathers are removed from commercially produced poultry by dipping the birds in mineral oil, another suspected cancer-causing agent. The only way to be sure you are avoiding these dangerous contaminants, as with buying eggs, is to locate a grower who raises poultry without the use of chemicals in the feed or in the process of preparing the poultry for market. We are sorry to add that packages of "chicken parts" are to be avoided. These "parts" are often removed from diseased birds, the rest going into pet food. By all means buy *whole* chickens and turkeys, because at least they will have been inspected for cancerous growths.

EVEN SOME FISH NOW CONTAMINATED

Fish. An ideal source of protein, fish are also generally low in fat. In addition to the nutrients they have in common with meat and poultry, many fish are also a good source of calcium, iron, and vitamin A. Because fish swim about feeding themselves, they are not contaminated with chemicals deliberately introduced into their diet by man. However, with the spread of pollution into our lakes, rivers, and oceans, pesticides are showing up in inland fish, and industrial wastes are being found even in deep-ocean fish. Water pollution is threatening the once plentiful populations of lobster, salmon, and crabs, and oil spills are depositing cancer-inducing hydrocarbons in microscopic marine organisms eaten by other organisms, moving up the food chain and eventually reaching the fish we eat and man himself. Mercury contamination of tuna and swordfish is a serious and controversial problem.

Because of all these possible sources of contamination, the safest kind of fish to eat is ocean fish. Since the level of pollution is lower in the open ocean, flounder, haddock, perch, sole, and other ocean fish are generally safer than the inland types. The flavor of fresh-caught fish is greatly superior to that of frozen and thawed fish. Avoid preserved or smoked fish (such as lox), which may contain dangerous levels of nitrites and nitrates.

SOME CANNED FISH A GOOD BUY

Tuna, Salmon, and Sardines. One of the most economical and versatile of fish, tuna is a great favorite with children. It contains over 25 percent of high-quality protein, and is one of the most protein-rich fish. Canned salmon is a good source of calcium when the soft bones are eaten, which is also true of sardines when eaten whole.

SHELLFISH RICH IN MINERALS

Shellfish. Oysters are an excellent source of calcium (94 mg. per 100 grams), being better in this regard than beef, lamb, and poultry. Zinc, often deficient in our diets, is gained by eating oysters. Remember, though, that oysters and some other shellfish are periodically infected with microbes transmitted by certain algae they eat; the characteristic color of these algae accounts for the name "red tide" that is applied to this condition in our coastal shellfish beds. Poisonings, sometimes fatal, have resulted from eating shellfish during these red tides, and for this reason you must be very sure of the source of your oysters, mussels, and other shellfish, and never collect them yourself during periods when government agencies have posted warnings of contaminated waters.

Other shellfish, also, are surprisingly nutritious. For example, crab meat contains an astonishing 2170 International Units (IUs) of vitamin A, while beefsteak contains about 20 IUs. Iodine, often deficient in most diets, is also found in fish, including shellfish.

SOME CHILDREN ALLERGIC TO SHELLFISH

One further warning is in order concerning shellfish. Many young children are hypersensitive to the protein in such shellfish as crabs and oysters, and particular care must be exercised with allergy-prone youngsters to introduce such foods in small quantities initially, until tolerance is known.

FRESH FISH LACK UNPLEASANT SMELL

That Fishy Smell. Children often "hate fish" because of the "fishy" smell. What causes this odor is that fish struggle before they die, the glycogen is depleted from their muscles, and lactic acid is not formed to act as a preservative. Another factor is the presence of a nitrogenous compound that is broken down by bacteria into trimethylamine, noted for its foul odor. The staler a fish is, the worse it smells, so your child may be intuitively correct in avoiding anything that "smells fishy."

A RECIPE FOR DISDAINERS OF SEAFOOD

A good recipe for fresh ocean fish is the following. Heat a bit of hot oil (olive), add fish, sauté only a few minutes on each side, turn, add chopped parsley, minced garlic, squeezed lemon juice, and *red* wine, to color the fish medium red. Turn, repeat seasonings, and sauté 3–5 minutes.

Of course, countless fish-stew recipes abound. We include the above recipe because it is so popular with the Weiner childen, who usually reject anything that swims.

RAW FISH A JAPANESE FAVORITE

You can also do what the Japanese have done since antiquity. Buy *fresh* raw fish (tuna, sea bass, etc.), slice it, and serve it with soy sauce. It is tasty and more nutritious than cooked fish, because the enzymes and vitamins have not been destroyed by heat.

MEAT, POULTRY, FISH, SHOPPING TIPS

Buying, Storing, and Cooking Meats, Poultry, and Fish. In addition to the cautions we've already given, remember that wrappers in the meat department can conceal a multitude of defects. You can't smell spoilage through a wrapper; nor can you see what the underside of that fresh-looking piece of meat looks like. Never buy meat in a damaged container, and avoid pieces of meat that have been marked down; there's a reason they are being sold at "bargain" prices, and it's probably not in the interest of your family's health. Your best assurance of good quality in meat is to have the butcher cut it fresh for you. Fresh meats are preferable to canned or packaged meats and are also less expensive; compare the price of a precooked ham with a fresh ham, for example. When you do buy processed meats, be sure to avoid those containing harmful preservatives such as nitrites, nitrates, and sodium erythrobate.

Vegetables

ROOT VEGETABLES STORE ENERGY AND VITAMINS THROUGH LEAN TIMES

The cultivation of vegetables has a long history, going back for some species as far as 7000 B.C. Vegetables supply us with many important vitamins and minerals. Root vegetables are also generally high in calories in the form of carbohydrates, and are used as staple foods in many cultures. Besides carbohydrates, the root vegetables also supply other valuable nutrients. White potatoes contain vitamin C and iron, while the yellow root vegetables such as carrots, yams, and sweet potatoes contain vitamin A. Well adapted to storing, root vegetables will keep through the winter, so they provide a good source of nutrients especially during times when fresh crops are not readily available.

LEGUMES RICH IN PROTEIN

Another group of vegetables, the legumes, including peas, beans, and lentils, are a good source of protein, although with the exception of those of the soybean they are *not* complete proteins. The legumes are of additional value because their roots have nodules that help to put nitrogen back into the ground; therefore they enrich the soil at the same time that they provide a valuable food.

Vegetables are also an important source of dietary fiber, valuable for keeping children "regular" while reducing their risk of developing appendicitis.

VEGETABLES SPRAYED, WAXED, DYED

Chemical Contamination of Vegetables. Unfortunately, we are likely to encounter some of the same problems with chemical contaminants in vegetables that we did with fruits. In recent years federal agencies have begun to respond to evidence of the dangers of pesticides by regulating some of the chemicals sprayed on vegetables, but we still have a long way to go to be sure that these harmful substances don't end up in the food we eat. Some farmers now grow vegetables naturally without pesticides, and you may be able to find such organically grown produce in health-food stores.

Besides the use of pesticides, vegetables are subjected to other chemical treatments of highly questionable safety. Potatoes, for example, are sometimes dyed red to make them appear new. In the past, sweet potatoes were dyed to make them look like the more expensive yams. Following the lead of Canada, this country effectively banned this practice in 1968 when the FDA forbade the interstate shipment of dyed potatoes—one of the rare instances in which artificial dyes have been prohibited in our foods.

Some root and bulb vegetables, such as potatoes, onions, and carrots, may sprout if they are stored for a long period of time. To prevent sprouting, which shortens their keeping life, they are treated with chemical inhibitors. One such substance, maleic hydrazide, has been shown to produce cancer in laboratory animals, and yet the use of potentially carcinogenic sprouting inhibitors continues. Even if vegetables are peeled, there is a chance that the chemical may have penetrated the skin, contaminating the flesh within. To test your supply of potatoes, onions, garlic, etc., store a few in a dark place, and if they begin to sprout, it is a sign that maleic hydrazide has *not* been used. The store where you bought them will then be a safe place to find your root crops.

MYSTERY OF TASTELESS TOMATOES UNRAVELED

Tomatoes are one of the most notorious disappointments in the modern supermarket. How often have we bought a nice, red, round tomato only to discover that it has no flavor at all? The reason for this is that tomatoes are picked when they are green, and then sprayed with ethylene to hasten the "ripening" process. Tomatoes are often also waxed to make them shiny and to keep them from bruising or shriveling. Obviously, vine-ripened tomatoes are vastly preferable to these tasteless impostors, but it's becoming increasingly difficult to find such tomatoes in the market.

Raw Vegetables and Salads. One of the best ways to eat vegetables is raw. Not only is the crisp, crunchy texture of raw vegetables appealing to the senses, but, even more important, cooking of any kind will almost always destroy some of the vitamin content of these nutritious foods. Vitamin C, which is abundant in many vegetables, is particularly susceptible to destruction through cooking.

NUTRIENTS ABOUND IN DARK-GREEN LEAVES

Salads offer a way of combining a number of healthful vegetables in almost unlimited ways. The green leafy vegetables used in salads have many benefits. To begin with, they are an important source of dietary fiber. In addition, green leafy vegetables contain an extremely wide variety of vitamins and minerals, including vitamins A, C, E, K, many B's, and iron, copper, magnesium, calcium, and other minerals, while they are very low in calories. An important point to remember is that it is the very green outer leaves that contain the highest concentrations of these important nutrients, while the blanched, whitish inner leaves, which many people favor in their salads, are actually much less rich in nutritional value. So don't throw away those nutrient-rich outer leaves when you make your salads! When they're left on lettuce and other greens, those outer leaves even allow the vegetables to continue increasing in vitamin content until wilting sets in.

Your salad will usually contain other highly nutritious raw vegetables as well, such as peppers, one of the richest known sources of vitamin C (especially when they ripen and turn red), and tomatoes, which supply vitamins A and C.

SPROUTS ADD INTEREST TO MANY DISHES

Sprouts. You are probably familiar with the bean sprouts used in Chinese food, which come from the sprouting of mung-bean seeds; but if you have never experimented with the sprouts of other seeds, such as alfalfa, cress, or radish, you are in for a tasty and highly nutritious surprise. Fresh sprouts are truly a "living food." Many markets are now carrying alfalfa sprouts as well as the more familiar mung-bean sprouts, but you can grow these and a wide assortment of other sprouts at home as well. Whether used to put the finishing touches on a salad or included as a crisp addition to a lunchtime sandwich, sprouts add another dimension to the sensory interest and healthfulness of many meals. Book IV contains complete instructions for sprouting seeds, beans, and grains in the "Miscellaneous" section of recipes.

FREEZING PRESERVES NUTRIENTS IN VEGETABLES

Preserving Vegetables. As we've already seen, the best way to eat most vegetables is fresh and uncooked. But when fresh vegetables aren't available, frozen vegetables are a good second choice. Modern freezing methods permit most vegetables to retain their nutrient value. In fact, some frozen vegetables may be fresher than the produce in the store; if they were flash-frozen right after harvest, they may have lost fewer vitamins than they would have during shipping to the market. However, as soon as frozen vegetables begin to thaw, they lose their nutrients more quickly than fresh vegetables, so you should follow the instructions on frozen vegetables and cook them while they're still frozen.

CANNED VEGETABLES CONTAIN SUGAR AND SALT

Canned vegetables retain much less of their nutrient value than fresh or frozen vegetables, and in addition they may have been chemically treated in the course of processing. If you read the labels on canned vegetables, you will discover that they often contain a great deal of added sugar and salt, neither of which is of any benefit in our already salt- and sugar-rich diets.

STEAMED VEGETABLES NEXT BEST TO FRESH

Cooking Vegetables. If raw vegetables are best, then steaming is generally the cooking method least likely to destroy nutrients. Boiling, on the other hand, generally produces a very nutritious pot of water while the vegetables lose their nutrients in equal measure. Quick stir-frying in a wok or frying pan, with a very small amount of unsaturated oil to help "seal in" the nutrients, is becoming another popular method for cooking vegetables, and a good way to preserve nutrient qualities. Refer to the "Vegetables" section of Book IV for other valuable tips in cooking vegetables.

ANIMAL PRODUCTS SUPPLY ALL ESSENTIAL AMINO ACIDS

Vegetarian Diets. With increasing population pressures and dwindling food supplies, more and more of the world's people are going to be relying on nonanimal sources for the proteins their bodies require. Proteins are made up of twenty-two amino acids, of which eight cannot be maufactured by our bodies. These eight are known as "essential amino acids" because they must be obtained from our food. Since protein is the material used to build and repair body cells, it is extremely important that we take in complete protein, which contains all eight essential amino acids. Animal products, including meat, poultry, fish, eggs, milk, and dairy products, contain complete protein, while most vegetable sources supply incomplete protein.

SOYBEAN THE ONLY VEGETABLE SOURCE
OF COMPLETE PROTEIN

The only exception is the soybean, which has long been recognized as capable of supporting life in the same way that animal products do. A staple in the Chinese diet for thousands of years, the soybean has demonstrated remarkable versatility eaten fresh; dried and stored; made into flour; used to make oil and even soy milk. The peanut is another good source of protein, although it is not quite a complete protein. Actually a pulse or legume rather than a nut, the peanut can support growth and maintenance of life but not reproduction. Whole grains are another source of incomplete protein.

VEGETABLE PROTEIN COMPLEMENTATION REQUIRED

Vegetable sources of incomplete protein can be combined in certain ways so that the amino acids provided by one complement the amino acids in another, with the combination supplying the complete protein required to sustain human life. Many cultures of the world have developed traditional combinations of protein-rich vegetables, intuitively developing diets that supply complete proteins. For example, whole-grain rice combined with beans supplies all essential amino acids.

There are many types of vegetarian diets, and it is certainly possible to obtain all the necessary nutrients on such diets. In addition, it is also a much more efficient way of using the nutrients available to us, since there is a tremendous loss of energy value when plant foods are fed to animals in order to produce calories in the form of meat, when the same plants might be eaten directly by humans.

SAFE VEGETARIAN DIET FOR CHILDREN OUTLINED

In spite of the undoubted value of many vegetarian diets, there is only one type that can be recommended for children. Known as the "*lacto-ovo-vegetarian* diet," it includes egg and dairy products as well as vegetable foods, thereby guaranteeing that complete proteins and other important nutrients will be available in the diet. In this diet, we must be sure to complement the protein sources to ensure an adequate supply of all the essential amino acids, through the correct combination of legumes, grains, and vegetables. The diet must also include milk, cheese, and eggs, since they supply vitamins B_{12} and A and minerals such as calcium and iron, as well as assuring a supply of all the important amino acids. The diet must also provide adequate folacin and zinc, which are sometimes lacking in vegetarian diets; and iodized salt or sea salt should be used (the relationship between salt and hypertension is amplified on page 127).

The dangers of serious nutritional deficiencies from some vegetarian regimens are too great for us to recommend this form of eating for all children. But most Americans today eat much more animal protein than they need, and there is some evidence that too much protein may be harmful, although probably not as harmful as too little. To help you get away from the daily routine of meat and potatoes, Book IV provides a number of meatless main dishes, using vegetable-protein sources such as legumes, grains, and nuts.

Starchy Staples

STARCHY FOODS PROVIDE CALORIES

Throughout the world, starchy staple foods form the basis of many widely varied diets. High in carbohydrates, these foods provide needed calories in areas where food supplies may otherwise be limited. They generally store well and thus serve to tide communities over during the hard winter months or periods of drought. Even in the United States, where we have a variety of sources of protein, vitamins, minerals, and calories, starchy foods are a traditional element of most dinners. While whole grains, root vegetables, wholesome breads, and other high-carbohydrate foods can be nourishing elements of a well-balanced diet, we must guard against the habitual compulsion to feed our children starchy foods that are devoid of much nutritional value other than their caloric content.

BROWN RICE A NUTRITIOUS STAPLE

Grains. While many grains and cereals are primarily used to make breads, some are eaten cooked as an accompaniment to meals, or as the basis of whole meals in themselves (see recipes in Book IV). Probably the most familiar example is *rice,* which is a staple food for hundreds of millions of people on our planet. Like whole-grain, unprocessed wheat, natural brown rice is a nutritious food, containing in its husk essential oils that are rich in B vitamins, and bran, among other nutrients. However, because its oil will become rancid, brown rice does not store well and is therefore milled, removing the nutrient-rich outer husks and leaving mainly starch. In this pure-white, devitalized form, rice will keep indefinitely. The by-products of the milling process are a source of extra profits for the food industry, the rice bran and rice polish being used in animal feeds and the rice oil becoming an ingredient in soaps and hair tonics.

Converted rice looks similar to white rice and cooks in the same way, but in fact it is far superior in nutritional value to white rice. To make converted rice, the whole, unmilled grains are treated with steam and pressure, dissolving the B vitamins and driving them into the center of the grain, where they are retained.

Brown rice, however, is by far the preferable form. It does take longer to cook than white rice, but its chewy texture and nutlike flavor are more than adequate compensation for the slight additional work it requires to prepare.

Some wheat products are also eaten as cooked grains, such as *bulgur wheat* and *cracked wheat;* see "How to Cook Cereals" in the Breakfast section of Book IV.

ETHNIC COMBINATION OF CORN AND BEANS SUSTAINS LIFE

Of course, *corn* is another widely used grain. North Americans are most accustomed to eating corn on the cob or as cornmeal, while in Mexico corn, in the form of tortillas, is part of a carefully balanced combination of vegetable protein sources. The combination of corn and beans provides all the essential amino acids needed to sustain life. In Europe, another cooked cornmeal product known as *polenta* serves as a starchy base for many meat and vegetable dishes.

Sorghum is the most important grain cereal in Africa. It somewhat resembles corn but is higher in protein and lower in fat. It is usually made into a meal, and is also used to make oil. A sweet sorghum variety in the United States is used to make a syrup.

Buckwheat, most familiar to us as an ingredient of pancakes, is a good source of B vitamins. In Eastern Europe it is used to make a cooked dish called *kasha,* which has sustained many generations of poor people. *Millet,* a cereal grass, is eaten both as a cereal and as a vegetable. Although it is mainly used for birdseed and pasturage in this country, it is a popular cooked dish in the Middle East. It contains trace amounts of amygdalin, the same reputed anticancer compound found in Laetrile.

You can obtain some of these less familiar grains, and some ethnic cereal products made from them, at health-food stores. You might want to try them as a change from the usual rice, potatoes, and bread by experimenting with the recipes in Book IV.

WHOLE-WHEAT NOODLES RECOMMENDED

Pasta. Ever since Marco Polo brought the trick of making flour into noodles from China to Europe, pasta has been a popular source of carbohydrates in the Western diet. While spaghetti, macaroni, and various forms of noodles can be made from a variety of grains, we are most familiar with those made from white flour. There are more nutritious pastas made from whole-wheat flour, or with spinach added, and spaghetti, being one of childhood's favorite dishes, should *always* be made from whole-wheat noodles, which are increasingly available.

POTATO AN IDEAL CHILDREN'S FOOD

Root Vegetables. Undoubtedly the most important tuber or root crop in the Western world is the potato, which has served as a staple food since the Spanish brought it back from the Andes of South America. This gift of South American Indian ingenuity soon became so successful a food that it made the eighteenth-century population explosion in Europe possible. A good source of vitamin C, iron, and protein, the potato is an ideal starchy vegetable for children. Remember to cook potatoes in their skins, and to serve them in ways that permit the skins to be eaten, since much good food fiber and minerals are contained in them. Some cases of severe malnutrition among children who cannot digest milk and dairy are treated successfully with potatoes, which provide a high-quality, digestible protein.

Other starchy root vegetables are important staples in other parts of the world. The cassava plant, for example, is the source of tapioca, an easily digested starchy food that can be used in puddings, bread, and as a thickening agent. Another tropical tuber, the taro root, is used to make the Polynesian staple known as *poi,* and is even eaten like the potato in Japan.

CARBOHYDRATES CONSTITUTE HALF OF CHILD'S DIET

The Role of Carbohydrates in Your Child's Diet. Besides starchy foods, sugars are also a source of carbohydrates in your child's diet, and, taken all together, carbohydrates should supply about half of the caloric intake. In general, starchy foods are less likely than sugars to cause digestive problems arising from irritation, fermentation, or early satiety. Table 8 lists common dietary sources of carbohydrates, with the foods grouped according to their carbohydrate content, from lowest to highest.

TABLE 8
Carbohydrate Content of Common Foods*
(Grouped according to percentage
of carbohydrate content)

5%	10%	20%	30%
Tomatoes	Pineapple	Ice cream	Peanuts
Pumpkin	Strawberries	Grapes	Coconut
Cauliflower	Peaches	Bananas	Chocolate
Cabbage	Oranges	Prunes	Sweet potatoes
Rhubarb	Lemons	Plums	Soybeans
	Grapefruit	Macaroni,	
	Apples	cooked	
	Apricots	Corn	
	Beets	Lima beans	
	Carrots	Potatoes	
	Turnips		
	String beans		

40%	60%	80%	100%
Bread:	Bread:	Rice	Milk sugar
corn	rye	Puffed rice	Cane sugar
whole wheat	wheat	Corn starch	Brown sugar
Cocoa	Oatmeal, dry	Barley	Candy
Chestnuts	Macaroni, dry	Shredded wheat	Dextrose
	Beans, dry	Tapioca	
	Macaroons	Figs	
	Molasses	Dates	
	Maple syrup	Honey	
		Maple sugar	

*After Kugelmass (1946).

PROPER ORDER FOR SERVING VEGETABLES AND SWEETS

In order to discourage excessive intake of sugars at the expense of more nutrient-rich high-carbohydrate foods, you should always offer vegetable and grain products *first* at a meal, reserving the sweets for last. Your child must be given the foods she likes least before the ones she craves.

Seasonings

SALT COMMON, BUT PRIZED

Salt. Used as a seasoning agent in foods since man's earliest days, salt is one of the commonest chemical compounds on the earth, yet because it is not evenly distributed on our planet, there has always been a lucrative trade in transporting salt from one place to another. The great caravan routes of the Sahara were largely for transporting salt, and whole empires were built upon trading salt from the north of the desert for the gold that lay to the south. The salt we use in our food is derived from mineral deposits of rock salt in the earth, as well as extracted from seawater. Besides being used to flavor foods, salt has also served the important function of acting as a preservative because it speeds the drying of foods and helps prevent discoloration and bacterial and mold growth.

NO NEED TO ADD SALT TO FOOD

Our palates have become so accustomed to the flavor of salt that we are now using far too much of it in our diet. In recent years it has become very clear that excess salt in the diet can cause high blood pressure and related diseases such as cerebrovascular disorders, even in children. Salt increases the body's ability to retain fluids, which is one reason why it aggravates high blood pressure. While it is undeniably true that salt is an essential nutrient for proper bodily functioning, we need only about one gram per day to meet our biological needs. This amount can be provided adequately by the foods we eat, and so we really do not need to add salt to our meals (the average American consumes about three grams a day).

SALT, STROKES, AND DEATH IN JAPAN

In a milestone study, N. Sasaki, M.D., reported on "The Relationship of Salt Intake to Hypertension in the Japanese" in 1964. He was convinced that the extraordinarily high incidence of death from apoplexy (stroke) in his country was related to dietary salt intake. Young adults without atherosclerosis die regularly from apoplexy in districts where food is pickled in brine. In fact, in one northeastern area of Japan, the Akita prefecture, a farming region that prides itself on its indigenous recipes for pickled vegetables, the blood pressures were higher than normal; and where the blood pressures were higher, so too was the mortality from apoplexy.

When you consider that we need only 1 gram of salt per day for survival, it is astounding to learn that the average resident of this region of Japan takes 27 grams a day! In regions where *less* salt is consumed, the mortality from apoplexy is also lower.

Now, it is true that the Japanese eat much vegetable food (rich in potassium), and so may crave salty seasonings such as miso, soy souce, pickles, etc., to get sodium for balance. But where people did *not* have inordinate cravings for salt, the blood-pressure levels and rates of death from apoplexy were lower (as in the Aomori prefecture, where the people eat many apples, which contain abundant amounts of potassium without inducing a craving for sodium).

SALT AN ACQUIRED TASTE

It has been observed that the taste for salt is acquired, and furthermore that we develop a tolerance to it. The more salt we eat in our food, the more we require in order to taste it; for this reason, it is essential that we avoid overly salty food in our children's diet, so that they do not become "salt addicts" at an early age, with increased risk of vascular disease later in life.

Commercially manufactured table salt contains chemical additives to protect it against moisture. To avoid these chemicals it is preferable to use unrefined sea or rock salt. These products are rich in minerals, but we should still use them in only very limited quantities.

SEA SALT A SOURCE OF NEEDED IODINE

Most commercial table salt is also iodized; that is, iodine has been added because in some parts of the country thyroid disease occurs as a result of a shortage of iodine in the soil and hence in crops grown in it. If we use sea salt, which contains iodine, this problem is solved without our having to consume the extra chemicals that are added to salt along with the iodine.

PEPPER NOT ESSENTIAL TO DIET

Pepper. The other very familiar seasoning on our dinner table is pepper. Unlike salt, this spice is not an essential element of the diet. Black pepper consists of the dried unripe berry of a tropical plant, while white pepper comes from the seed inside the berry. Like many other spices, pepper has traditionally been used not only as a flavoring agent for food but also as a medicine. It has been considered good for the digestion and has been used to induce fever. It is best avoided by children except in some cases of constipation, in which its stimulating properties on the bowels are valuable. (Cayenne pepper, another species, is excellent for stubborn cases of constipation.)

SPICES FORMERLY USED TO DISGUISE SPOILED FOODS

Other Spices. Spices may be defined as vegetable products that are used to flavor foods, which derive their pungent or aromatic qualities from the essential oils they contain. Generally, the part of the plant containing the highest concentration of these oils is the part used as a spice. In the past, before the introduction of modern refrigeration methods, spices were used to conceal the taste and odor of spoiled food. Many spices have also been used as medicines. Because most spices grew in remote tropical countries far from the European market that craved them, these flavoring agents were very highly prized and formed the basis of a rich trade that created fortunes for entire countries.

Besides pepper, some of the most widely used spices today are described below.

Cinnamon is derived from the inner bark of an evergreen tree that is native to Ceylon. The essential oil is used medicinally for stomach complaints. *Cloves* are the dried buds of another evergreen tree grown in the West Indies, Zanzibar, and the Molucca Islands. Oil of cloves is a common household remedy for toothache, and is also used medicinally as an antispasmodic. *Nutmeg* is the fruit of an evergreen tree that grows in the West Indies. The fruit actually contains two spices, a fiber within the husk that is known as "mace" and the actual nutmeg inside the mace. Nutmeg and its oil have been used as an insomnia remedy, a stimulant, and a flavoring agent for medicines; and apiol, one of the constituents of nutmeg oil, is used for kidney problems. (Nutmeg in large quantities is toxic!) *Mace* contains among its essential oils a substance known as myristicin, which in large quantities can cause liver damage.

HERBS AS FOOD, MEDICINE, FLAVORING

Herbs. Herbs may be broadly defined as any plants useful to man. In cooking they usually consist of the herbaceous or green and flowering parts of a nonwoody plant. Used to flavor foods and sometimes to enhance their appearance, many herbs also have medicinal properties, and some supply important nutrients as well. There is sometimes an unclear line separating herbs from vegetables, since some herbs, especially green leafy ones, can also be used, for example, as salad greens. In general, culinary herbs are used in such small quantities as seasonings that their contribution to the nutrient content of food is negligible. However, some are so rich in nutrients that they can make a significant contribution to any dish they are used in. Parsley, for example, is extremely rich in vitamin A, as well as containing vitamin C, iron, and other minerals. Paprika, a source of vitamin A, is reputed to be good for night vision, and it also supplies vitamin C, even in powdered form. Other herbs that will enliven your cooking include basil, bay leaf, chervil, chives, dill, marjoram, oregano, peppermint, rosemary, sage, tarragon, and thyme. They can be used to create new interest in vegetable dishes, soups, meats, fish, poultry, and eggs, in virtually unlimited combinations.

USE ONLY NATURAL FLAVORS

Extracts and Artificial Flavors. Another way of adding flavor to foods, especially desserts and baked goods, is through the use of extracts, which are generally alcohol solutions of the essential oils of natural vegetable products, such as vanilla, almond, mint, or lemon. (Note: some children are allergic to alcohol in *any* form, even in the small amounts present in extracts.) However, there is a great tendency today to use the much cheaper and more potent artificial flavors instead of these natural products.

Many of these artificial flavors are made from chemical compounds known to be dangerous to the health, including coal-tar derivatives, allergens, irritating substances, and narcotics. Artificial flavors and colors are also suspected to contribute to hyperactivity in children. These harmful chemical substances are used in all sorts of processed foods, particularly pastries, ice cream, soft drinks, and other foods largely aimed at our youngsters. There is no reason to expose our children to the dangers of these substances, and we should always check the labels on packaged foods to be sure that they contain no artificial flavors or colors.

MSG COMMON IN PROCESSED FOODS

Monosodium Glutamate. Probably the most commonly used flavoring agent in our foods today is monosodium glutamate, or MSG. This so-called flavor enhancer actually works by stimulating the response of our taste buds so that the food, which may be overly processed and lacking in flavor, is made to appear to have a taste that it doesn't. This is obviously a rather roundabout way of making food taste good. In experimental animals (infant mice) MSG in high doses has been shown to cause brain damage. MSG is widely used in Chinese restaurants, and some individuals who are sensitive to this chemical develop an allergic reaction to it consisting of a tightness about the jowls and occasionally dizziness, headache, weakness, and malaise, all known as the "Chinese-restaurant syndrome." (Incidentally, many Chinese restaurants will now serve food without MSG when specifically requested to do so. Just say *"No may gin"* when ordering your meal, if you suspect your waiter doesn't understand "MSG." While there should be little temptation to add this product to your cooking at home (even in Chinese recipes, which almost routinely call for it), it is quite difficult to avoid it in processed foods, and so once again it is only through a careful reading of the labels that we can avoid another source of chemical tampering with our children's diet.

Oils

FAT REDUCTION BENEFITS ALL DIETS

Saturated and Unsaturated Fats. It has been demonstrated in recent years that the consumption of large quantities of saturated fats in the diet can lead to excess cholesterol in the blood. This elevated cholesterol level can in turn contribute to atherosclerotic heart disease.

TABLE 9
Fat Content of Common Foods*
(Grouped according to percentage
of fat content)

10%	20%	30%	40%
Cookies	Veal	Pork	Cream (heavy)
Crackers	Beef	Lamb	Peanuts
Zwieback	Fowl	Egg yolk	
Oatmeal	Fish (canned)	Coconut	
Chicken	Cream (light)	Cocoa	
Brain	Olives	Cream cheese	
Eggs	Avocado		
Evaporated Milk	Soybeans		
Ice cream			

50%	60%	85%	100%
Peanut butter	Bacon	Butter	Halibut-liver
Almonds	Walnuts	Oleomargarine	oil
Chocolate	Butternuts		Cod-liver oil
	Brazil nuts		Corn oil
			Olive oil
			Cottonseed oil

*After Kugelmass (1946).

For this reason, it has been recommended that people switch from saturated to unsaturated fats in their diet, and that they also lower their total fat intake. Although these dietary recommendations are aimed primarily at adults, it is beneficial to avoid excessive fats, particularly saturated fats, in our children's diet as well, and so we should avoid fatty meats and greasy foods cooked in saturated fats. Table 9 lists the fat content of common foods, in increasing order of fat content.

COCONUT AND CHOCOLATE HIGH IN SATURATED FAT

The degree of saturation of a fat is determined by the number of hydrogen atoms attached to the carbon atoms in its molecules; if all available carbon bonds are taken up by hydrogen atoms, the fat is said to be saturated, while in an unsaturated fat some of the carbon bonds are not attached to hydrogen molecules. In general, the more solid a fat is, the more saturated it is. Animal fats, which are usually solid at room temperature, are generally highly saturated, while vegetable and fish oils are generally unsaturated. Important exceptions are coconut oil and chocolate, two plant fats that are both highly saturated. Unfortunately, coconut oil is fairly inexpensive and is therefore often used for deep-frying, as well as for making baked goods, imitation milks, candies, and other processed foods.

UNSATURATED OILS ADVISED FOR COOKING

Unsaturated vegetable oils, made from seeds, nuts, and legumes such as soy, safflower, peanut, sesame, corn, and sunflower, can be used in baking, in salad dressings, and as cooking agents for frying. They are the source of important nutrients such as linoleic acid, an essential fatty acid and should be included in any child's diet. However, since fats are generally overconsumed in the

United States, the recipes in Book IV are all prepared without the use of oils or fats of any kind.

SHORTENING A HIGHLY PROCESSED FAT

Hydrogenation. In order to increase the shelf life of unsaturated oils and to facilitate their handling, the food industry has developed a process known as hydrogenation, whereby unsaturated oils are changed into hard, saturated oils through a process of heating and the introduction of hydrogen under pressure in the presence of a catalyst. As the hydrogen forms bonds with the unsaturated carbon atoms in the oil, the oil becomes hard. The resulting product is then bleached, and any taste and odor are eliminated through chemical processing. Needless to say, this hydrogenated fat has been robbed of all the valuable vitamins, minerals, and essential fatty acids that were present in the original oil, leaving behind nothing but calories. Hydrogenated fats are commonly called for in recipes in the form of "shortening"—for example, in baked goods. It is always preferable to use wholesome butter or unsaturated oils for such purposes.

WHY TO AVOID MARGARINE

Margarine. A particularly worthless hydrogenated fat, margarine should never be used as a substitute for butter in your child's diet. Although some margarines are advertised as being high in unsaturates, this claim is really meaningless since the margarine wouldn't be solid at room temperature if it didn't contain at least some hydrogenated fats. The artificial butter flavor and odor in these products comes from diacetyl, a derivative of the toxic chemical butanol. Also added are artificial color, preservatives that are known to produce illness in some people, and synthetic vitamins. It is a sad commentary on the ethics of our food industry that the American anxiety about heart disease is exploited by replacing butter, a wholesome natural food (although it contains saturated fat), with a nonnutritious mixture of synthetic ingredients in the form of margarine, which contains a much more harmful kind of saturated fat and dangerous additives. Of course, margarine is cheaper than butter—as it should be, with its virtually nonexistent nutritional value—but this is no reason to use it in place of butter.

FRENCH FRIES CARRY HIDDEN CANCER RISK

Deep-frying. Children—and we parents as well—are very fond of "French"-fried potatoes and other foods fried in fat. Recently the National Cancer Institute has reported that cancer-producing substances can be formed through the repeated heating of hydrogenated fats, which are commonly used in commercial French-frying. For this reason, we must be careful to avoid foods that have been fried at high temperatures in fats that have been reused excessively. If the oil used for French-frying at a food stand looks brown or smells peculiar, don't buy their products, and never hesitate to ask how long the same oil has been in the French-fryer.

POTATO CHIPS HIGH IN FAT, SALT; LOW IN NUTRIENTS

As appealing as French-fried foods may be to the senses, they are not very nutritious. Not only are they often cooked in hydrogenated fat; they also lose most of their nutrients in the course of being cooked at high temperatures. Moreover, French-fried potatoes, for example, may have been treated with chemicals prior to cooking. Similarly, potato chips, another favorite food of children, are often cooked in rancid oils, and rancidity can cause the destruction of many vitamins. Of course, potato chips are also high in salt content, another good reason to omit them from your child's diet.

How Much to Eat?

LIGHT DINNER ADVISED

No matter how nutritious the food you provide for your child may be, it is important to guard against overeating. Some recent studies have implicated overeating as one of the major causes of a wide variety of disease. For this reason, dinner should be one of the *lightest* meals of the day, which will also make it easier for your child to sleep.

A good rule of thumb is to eat
¼ of the day's food for breakfast
½ of the day's food for lunch
¼ of the day's food for dinner.

During the summer, it may be better for the biggest meal to be taken in the evening, when the cooler temperatures are more conducive to proper digestion.

BEDTIME

Because the digestive system, along with all the other internal organs, needs to "rest" from its daytime functions during sleep, it is never a good idea for your child to eat significant quantities of food close to bedtime. One of the worst habits that can be acquired in childhood is to snack late in the evening; the food eaten late at night adds unnecessary calories, which can contribute to a lifelong problem with obesity.

However, certain light, nutritious foods, given in small quantities, may be appropriate as bedtime snacks. Especially valuable is milk; it may be given cold, and when served warm it has an age-old reputation for inducing restful sleep (because of its high tryptophan content).

BEVERAGES

*Stolen waters are sweet, and bread
eaten in secret is pleasant.*
PROVERBS 9:17

Water

WATER ESSENTIAL TO BODY PROCESSES

Biological Functions of Water. Even though water provides no nutrients except small quantities of minerals, it is one of the most important substances we consume in the course of our daily intake of food and drink. Water is absolutely essential for proper bodily function. Although people have reportedly gone without food for weeks, we can survive only a few days without water, for our bodies will become dehydrated and the fluid balance disrupted. Water serves as the vehicle for carrying nourishment to the body's cells and for carrying waste materials away; it is also the basis of the cooling system that keeps our temperature stable at 98.6°. It is a constituent of all the fluids secreted and excreted by our bodies.

You may wonder why doctors always advise us to drink plenty of fluids when we get sick. During times of fever or infection, we need extra fluids to circulate through our bodies, carrying away the toxic substances from our tissues and helping to reduce body temperature.

Water may also be a source of some valuable minerals. In areas where the water is "hard," it may contain calcium or magnesium salts.

The approximately 2½ quarts of water we require each day are provided not only in the form of beverages but also from the water content of our soups, fruits, vegetables, meat—in fact, everything we eat contains some water; but it is still important to be sure we drink enough fluids.

WATER SUPPLY CONTAMINATED

How Safe Is Tap Water? Considering how important water is to our health, we have due cause for alarm when we look at the quality of our modern water supply. Tap water in the United States today is of questionable safety. Through treatment with chlorine, dangerous bacteria such as those that cause typhoid and cholera are eliminated, but the chlorine itself may combine with other chemicals and produce carcinogenic compounds. Viruses may pass through filtration systems and produce epidemics of disease. Even more common is contamination from industrial waste; chemicals dumped into our air and our waterways may end up in the water we drink, along with petroleum products from oil spills. Such water-soluble compounds as benzene, ether, chloroform, and other organic materials are known to cause cancer; at present there are no purity standards protecting us against such substances in our water supply. In agricultural areas, pesticide residues in the soil enter the water table and end up in the water supply. In communities where lead pipes are used, the lead may enter the drinking water, and other communities have mercury, asbestos, copper, and other harmful materials in their drinking water as well.

FLUORIDATION LINKED TO CANCER

Fluoridation. For some years, fluoride has been added to the water supply in many communities as a preventive measure against dental caries. While there is little doubt that fluoride *does* prevent caries, there is also significant evidence linking water fluoridation with increased rates of cancer in the United States. While a recent study by Dr. Dean Burke, former director of the National Cancer Institute, shows a direct relationship between fluorides and carcinogenesis, medical and industrial "authorities" who repeat uncritically what they "have heard," or "understand," to be true continue to promote this dangerous practice. As the bumper sticker says, we should "fluoridate candy, *not* water!" Why put *all* age groups at risk with this questionable chemical when it reduces the risk of tooth decay only in the young?

WATER FILTER RECOMMENDED

Sources of Pure Water. Throughout human history, the safety of the community's water supply has been a concern of the highest priority. With all the new sources of contamination from modern industry, it will be some time before new purification methods are instituted to protect us against this modern chemical plague. In the meantime, it might be worth considering using a sink-top filtration unit for your drinking water, or buying only bottled spring water, provided that the "spring" is un-contaminated.

Milk

Next to plenty of pure water, the next most impor-tant beverage for your child is of course whole milk. (See page 87 for details.)

Fruit Beverages

FRESH-SQUEEZED JUICES BEST BY FAR

Juices. Real fruit juices, freshly squeezed from fresh, ripe fruits (and from some vegetables as well), contain the same nutrients as do the fruits themselves. (Remember, though, that the longer juice sits after squeezing, the greater is the nutrient loss.) A blender, or better yet a juicer, is a good investment for your home because it will allow you to extract juice from some fruits and vegetables that are difficult to squeeze by hand. Be sure to add some of the pulp to the juice, to benefit from the minerals, fiber, and bioflavonoids.

Next to fresh-squeezed juice the best thing is frozen fruit juice, in which most of the nutrients are preserved intact, while canned and bottled juices are slightly lower in nutritional value. Be very careful to read the label when you buy fruit juices, because you want to buy only those products that contain no added sugar. Such juices will be labeled "unsweetened" or "no sugar added."

Ades. Lemonade, orangeade, or limeade is another kind of fruit beverage that is very popular as a cooling summertime drink or throughout the year. Made from freshly squeezed fruit juice diluted with water and with sweetener added, these drinks are not as nutritious as undiluted fruit juices. Furthermore, they are usually sweetened with sucrose, and should be avoided for this reason.

WATER, SUGAR, CHEMICALS, POSE AS CHILDREN'S DRINK

"Fruit Drinks." Beware of the canned, bottled, or frozen beverages labeled "fruit drinks." While they may be adorned with tempting pictures of fruit, and while they may be a lot less expensive than fruit juice, these beverages really contain little but water, sugar, and artificial flavor and color. Be careful to inspect the label on any fruit beverage to make sure you are not wasting your money, and risking your child's health, on these nonnutritious products.

Soft Drinks

SODA POP HIGHLY DESTRUCTIVE

Even worse than these fruit drinks are the sodas or soft drinks that contain carbonation. Taking the harmful potential of fruit drinks a step further, these soft drinks contain acids that are strong enough to dissolve tooth enamel! The sugar in these drinks—usually about 5 teaspoons in an 8-ounce bottle!—provides a perfect setting for bacteria to reproduce in the mouth, and adds even more to the acid concentration already present in the soda. As with other sugary processed foods, soft drinks may actually induce protein deficiencies in youthful soft-drink "addicts" who don't take in enough nourishing food because the sugary drinks dull their appetite. In extreme cases, such adolescent "addicts" have developed cirrhosis of the liver. Dentists are well aware of the dangers of soft drinks, and frequently warn their young patients and their parents against them.

Besides the sugar and acid in soft drinks, there is little but a combination of chemicals, with no nutrients whatever except the empty calories of their sugar content. Cola drinks almost always contain caffeine, which can have powerful adverse effects on youngsters. The phosphoric acid present in colas also upsets the delicate calcium/phosphorus balance. Diet soft drinks contain saccharin instead of sugar; we have already seen that saccharin is a potentially dangerous substance.

Coffee and Tea, Caffeine

HERB TEAS OK; AVOID CAFFEINE

You might wonder whether it is wise to give your child coffee or tea. Caffeine, present in both these popular beverages, is a powerful central-nervous-system stimulant whose effects are even more pronounced in children, producing increased heartbeat and breathing rates. Some people value caffeine for its ability to keep them awake, but it can also cause insomnia, irregular heartbeat, nervousness, and even convulsions in very large doses. After drinking coffee or caffeine-containing cola, children often become hyperactive, restless, and unable to concentrate. Caffeine is also now suspected of being able to cause birth defects if consumed during pregnancy. Any substance that can produce such powerful adverse effects must be considered unfit for our children, and for these reasons coffee should not be given to them.

Black tea also contains caffeine. There are, however, many refreshing and tasty caffeine-free herb teas, such as chamomile, peppermint, lemon grass, and many popular blends that are now available. Remember that some of these herbs may have medicinal effects if taken in excessive quantities, so don't give them to your child until you have evaluated the contents of herbal-tea blends.

Chocolate

CAROB BETTER THAN CHOCOLATE

Chocolate comes from the cacao tree, an evergreen of the kola family. It doesn't contain caffeine, but it does contain another stimulant, theobromine, which has effects quite similar to those of caffeine. When used to make cocoa, the amount of theobromine present would be comparable to the caffeine in a cup of weak coffee or tea (approximately 30 mg.). Of course, chocolate is also a saturated fat and is high in calories, and when used in cocoa it is usually sweetened with sugar. Copper is also abundant in chocolate and must be avoided by "hyperactive" children who often have low zinc and high copper levels. For the same reasons, we *never* use cocoa or "hot chocolate" at home. They may seem innocent enough, but in fact are great nutritional time bombs filled with sucrose, bleaches, copper, artificial flavorings, and excess calories. Stick to warm milk flavored with carob powder and sweetened with honey, which makes a fine bedtime drink.

BOOK III
Natural Approaches for Natural Complaints

Disease! That is the main force, the diligent force, the devastating force! It attacks the infant the moment it is born; it furnishes it one malady after another: croup, measles, mumps, bowel troubles, teething pains, scarlet fever, and other childhood specialties. It chases the child into youth and furnishes it some specialties for that time of life. It chases the youth into maturity, maturity into age, and age into the grave.

MARK TWAIN, Letters from the Earth

VITAMIN C, PROTEIN, MUST BE EATEN

Amid all the furious debate and battling among the "experts" in nutrition, people somehow manage to feed themselves and survive, often on very little. How is it that some of us can eat foods containing less than the Recommended Dietary Allowances (RDAs) of various nutrients and yet manage to grow, and age? The skeptics would tend to think that we are highly adaptive organisms who can manufacture what we need from just about any combination of foods we choose. This is, of course, untrue. We cannot manufacture vitamin C from any other starting compounds: it *must* be supplied from our foods. And in the case of viral illness, large supplemental quantities are required to lessen the effects and to speed recovery. Certainly we cannot manufacture the essential amino acids from fats or carbohydrates; these protein "building blocks" must be derived from the foods we eat. Likewise with numerous nutrients, particularly the trace minerals (such as zinc, selenium, chromium, etc.), which tend to be in short supply in the diets of technological societies. These too must come from our foods; they cannot be manufactured from a helter-skelter conglomeration of fat- and sucrose-ridden "empty" diets.

SUPPLEMENT-POPPING HAS REPLACED PILL-POPPING

At the other extreme are the dietary neurotics who believe we are suffering from the diseases of civilization that can be prevented or eliminated only through the use of a variety of nutritional supplements. Touring a contemporary "health food" store, we are impressed by the wide array of pills being sold as supplements. People have justifiably lost faith in the synthetic drugs promulgated by physicians who have learned all the sciences of medicine except one: the art of healing. But now, replacing the antibiotics, cough medicines, aspirin, and tranquilizers are other bottled pills, albeit more "natural" because they are found in natural products. These vitamins, minerals, amino acids, enzymes, and glandular extracts do have a *limited* role in our health-maintenance programs, primarily when we are ill, or to augment deficient diets.

FOOD AS MEDICINE

FOOD THE OLDEST MEANS OF PREVENTION AND TREATMENT

Food remains our best medicine. It has been so since prehistory, and remains so in the age of cosmic exploration. We have traveled far from our planetary roots but remain physiologically identical to our prehistoric ancestors. What worked to prevent and treat illness then still works. It is simply a matter of knowing which foods to eat and which to withhold. With *minor* supplementation and appropriate herbal remedies as adjuncts, you should be able to treat your child adequately for most common complaints. (*Of course, should any symptoms persist, or where serious inflammation or fever is manifest, we strongly urge you to consult a competent pediatrician.* We hope someone who will encourage you to assist in your child's recovery.)

TIME-TESTED DIETS PROVIDED

The diets for disease states included in this section have been adapted from *The Newer Nutrition in Pediatric Practice*, by the eminent pediatrician Dr. I. N. Kugelmass (1940). Based upon thousands of clinical cases and widely used by the medical profession prior to the "antibiotic age," these regimens reflect the wisdom of the ages while utilizing contemporary foods. *Employed under the supervision of your pediatrician*, the diets in this section offer you the best approach to caring for an infant or a child who is *not* so seriously ill as to need hospitalization. By combining your physician's scientific tools and remedies with *your* loving art of feeding according to these "sickroom regimens," a practical synthesis of the art and the science of healing can be achieved.

THE ROLE OF VITAMIN/MINERAL SUPPLEMENTS IN CHILDHOOD ILLNESS

FOODS AND HERBS PREFERRED TO SUPPLEMENTS

You will *not* find radical suggestions here for using vitamins and minerals in treating your child at home. A general multivitamin/mineral formula, described in Appendix B, is suggested for use on a preventive basis, and a vitamin C/wheat-germ oil/grape-juice drink, appropriate for most viral illnesses, is described on page 147. But megadoses of nutrients for children are unwise, until more is known about their actions, fate, excretion routes, and *interactions* with one another, with drugs, and with foods.

There are books on childhood nutrition that prescribe alarmingly large dosages of most nutrients for all varieties of complaints, from autism to xenophobia! This approach is unwise, in our opinion, when the entire life cycle of your child is considered. Short-term results may be spectacular, while in the long term possible untoward results mitigate in favor of foods and herbal teas, both therapeutic modes having withstood the test of time. It

TABLE 10
Vitamin Dosage Reference Chart

Vitamin	RDA (Infants—Pregnancy)	SR (Supplement Range) (Infants—Adults)
A	2000–5000 IU	2000–20,000 IU
B_1	0.3–1.6 mg	10–100 mg
B_2	0.4–1.8 mg	10–100 mg
B_6	0.3–2.8 mg	10–100 mg
B_{12}	0.5–4.0 mcg	0.5–4.0 mcg
Biotin	none*	20–1000 mcg
Choline	none*	250 mg–1 gm
Folic Acid	30–800 mcg	30–1000 mcg
Inositol	none*	400 mg–several grams
Niacin	6–19 mg	50–100 mg
Pantothenic Acid	none*	50–100 mg
PABA	none*	50–500 mg
B_{15}	none*	10–150 mg
C	35–100 mg	50 mg–150 grams
D	200–400 IU	200–400 IU
E	3–11 mg	10–400 mg

*"None" does *not* mean that these nutrients are not required, but an RDA for these nutrients has not been established.

may well prove to be the case that our synthetic or extracted vitamin and mineral concentrates are not as valuable as these same vitamins and minerals in our food, since in natural sources they may occur with other, as yet unidentified trace substances that may greatly increase their effectiveness.

A VITAMIN-C PREPARATION FOR ILLNESS

A "COCKTAIL" FOR VIRAL DISEASES

A particularly fine tonic for times of illness consists of vitamin-C powder in a mixed form of ascorbic acid and sodium ascorbate, at the level of approximately ⅓ teaspoon or 2 grams, together with approximately 1 tablespoon of wheat-germ oil, which is sweet, all mixed in a glass of juice, such as grape juice. The sweet wheat germ, combined with the bitter vitamin-C powder and buffered by the juice, makes for a highly palatable sickbed tonic for children

DOSAGE OF VITAMIN C DEPENDS ON ILLNESS

How do we know how much vitamin C to give during the flu, colds, and other viral disorders? According to Dr. Cathcart, who has had great experience with administering this vitamin, we should give this nutrient up until the point at which diarrhea occurs, and then back it off 10 percent. He claims that the sicker we are, the more vitamin C we need and can therefore tolerate. And so, if you have been trying, let's say, 500 mg. or 1000 mg. of vitamin C for a cold or the flu, and have experienced no change in the illness, Dr. Cathcart tells us that you probably have a 3000 or a 10,000 or a 15,000 mg. viral disorder. So remember, if you try vitamin C and it doesn't "work," then try some more; but be sure to use the vitamin-C powder in a form that is balanced between ascorbic acid and sodium ascorbate to avoid diarrhea at a low dosage level, with about a tablespoonful of the recommended wheat-germ oil in a glass of juice.

HERBAL PREPARATIONS FOR CHILDHOOD COMPLAINTS

HERBS SAFE FOR CHILDREN OVER 2

In addition to the specialized diets for specific childhood complaints, we have provided some suggestions for herbal preparations that will be helpful for specific symptoms or for generalized illnesses. The dosages of these herbal remedies have been specifically adjusted for children from 2 to 12 years of age. For children over the age of 12, the adult dosage may be given, which is twice the amount of the herb with the same quantity of water. *For infants under 2, use herbs with extreme caution;* the infant's body utilizes and eliminates nutrients and medicines in a way different from the older child's, and some generally harmless herbs may cause problems for the tiniest babies. Certain herbal remedies, however, are appropriate even for infants, and we have indicated where specific herbal preparations are safe for this age group.

COMPLEX HERBAL FORMULAS MAY BE USED

For most disorders, we offer a selection of possible herbs you may choose from. For the sake of simplicity, we give directions for making preparations for only *single* herbs, rather than combinations.

ABOUT THE DIETS

REFINED CARBOHYDRATES HELPFUL IN ILLNESS

In the dietary treatments outlined in this section for various disorders, you will find some foods suggested that we would not recommend for the feeding of a healthy child, such as refined cereal gruels or cereal waters prepared from refined starches. During some childhood illnesses, digestive upset is such a problem that whole grains and other nutritious foods produce too much irritation to be tolerated. In such cases it is only by introducing calories in the form of refined carbohydrates that we can provide needed energy in the sick child's diet, helping to maintain strength during this period of stress.

Similarly, while it is not generally a good idea to add sweetener to your child's food when she is healthy, the use of added sweetener during illness may also serve to boost energy intake without disturbing a touchy digestive system.

BLACKSTRAP MOLASSES A HEALTHFUL ADDED SWEETENER

At the time Dr. Kugelmass wrote his landmark book on diets for disease states, there were a great many different sugars available for addition to infants' and children's feedings. Today, many of these often-useful sugars, such as dextrimaltose, are no longer available; and so in place of the various sugars recommended by Dr. Kugelmass we have substituted *blackstrap molasses*. If you will refer to Table 6, page 95, you will see how nutritious this unrefined product is compared to our usual refined sugars. Dr. Lester Luz, a San Francisco pediatrician, has been using blackstrap molasses successfully for over three decades, in all cases where children need additional quantities of absorbable sweetener. The quantity he recommends for addition to an infant's formula is a mere ¼ teaspoon per bottle.

HONEY TO BE USED WITH CAUTION

You may also choose to try using honey where an added sweetener is suggested in the diets, but you must keep two crucial points in mind. Honey is quite safe for normal children in moderate amounts, but it is capable of producing severe *allergic reactions* in susceptible children; so if your child has allergic tendencies, you must be very cautious about introducing honey into his diet. Secondly, *we must warn you against using raw honey for infants.* The use of raw honey has been implicated in some cases of sudden-infant-death syndrome, probably owing to the incubation of bacteria in honey to which infants, but not older children, are susceptible. If you give honey to your infant, be sure that it has been *boiled* to kill the bacteria that may live in the raw form of this nutritious food.

SPECIAL FOODS FOR THE SICKROOM

SICK CHILDREN NEED DIFFERENT FOODS

In some of the diets that follow, you will find references to special foods for feeding sick children. We provide the directions for preparing these foods here, as Kugelmass originally described them, but adapted to the selection of ingredients that are readily available today.

Starchy Foods

Thick Feedings. Milk mixtures may be thickened by the addition of flours; such thick foods are helpful in feeding vomiting patients because they cannot be forced up through the opening of the stomach.

You may prepare a thick feeding from breast milk or from whole, skimmed, or evaporated cow's or goat's milk. Do not use skim milk unless your child's problem is related to fat intolerance.

Make a smooth paste of barley or other flour by mixing with a small amount of the milk. Add the remaining milk, stirring constantly, while cooking over a low flame for about 15 minutes, or in a double boiler for about 30 minutes, until the mixture becomes thick. A small amount of sweetener may be added, and then the mixture divided into the number of bottles required and refrigerated. A large opening will be needed in the nipple to give a thick feeding from a bottle; older infants may be given the feeding by spoon.

Cereal Gruels

For most cereals, such as barley, farina, rice, etc., add ½ cup of cereal to 1 pint of boiling water. Cook over direct flame for 20 minutes, stirring vigorously to prevent lumping. A little salt may be added for flavor (unless contraindicated in a particular illness).

To make a *cereal jelly,* prepare the cereal as described above until thickened; then strain and pour into molds, and refrigerate.

Oatmeal gruel Add ¼ cup of oatmeal to 1½ cups of boiling water; cook 20 minutes, stirring frequently.

Cereal gruels or jellies may be kept refrigerated in a glass bowl for a day.

Cereal Waters

These are used in the treatment of diarrhea. To make *barley, oatmeal,* or *rice water,* wash, soak, and cook 1 tablespoon of the barley, oatmeal, or rice flour in 2 cups of water until the liquid is boiled down to 1 cup. Strain.

To make *arrowroot water,* make a paste consisting of 2 teaspoons of arrowroot powder and 2 tablespoons of cold water. Add 1 cup of boiling water and cook for 2 hours in a double boiler. Salt, if desired, and strain.

Other Cereal Recipes

For further general instructions on cooking cereals, refer to "How to Cook Cereals" in Book IV, page 280.

Acid Milks

Lactic-Acid Milk. While naturally fermented milks are generally best, in times of illness you may not have a cultured acid milk, such as yogurt or kefir, available. Or you may want to give your child an acidified milk prepared from a milk of your own choosing, such as skim or evaporated milk, or goat's milk.

In order to make lactic-acid milk at home, you will need to keep some lactic acid on hand; this is available at your pharmacy, in liquid form. Boil and cool the required amount of milk, then add lactic acid in the proportion of 1½ teaspoons to 1 quart of milk or 5 drops per ounce of milk. Add the lactic acid *drop by drop,* stirring constantly. This milk may be used instead of cultured fermented milks.

Lactic acid may also be added to unsweetened evaporated milk to which an equal quantity of water has been added, using 3 drops of lactic acid per ounce of milk, adding drop by drop and stirring constantly.

The enzyme *lactase* is also available commercially. For instructions on "predigesting" milk with this enzyme, see the final paragraph of the discussion under "Milk Intolerance" in this section, on page 242.

Protein Foods

Gelatin. Prepare *unflavored and unsweetened* gelatin according to the directions on the package, using fruit juice for flavoring and sweetening.

Junket. Dissolve one junket tablet by crushing it in a cup along with 1 tablespoon of *cold* water. Warm 1 quart of milk to about 98° F. and add a little fruit juice and a little sweetener (molasses or honey) if desired. Add the dissolved junket tablet to the milk mixture, stir, and pour into dessert glasses. Let stand until firm.

SICKROOM RECIPES NOT FOR THE HEALTHY

Remember that the foods described above are for use in time of illness; we do *not* recommend refined starches, skim or low-fat milk, or the habitual use of added sweetener in the diet of a normal, healthy child.

ACNE

Acne vulgaris, such a common source of embarrassment in puberty and adolescence, is a skin eruption arising from changes in the consistency of the fatty secretions of the sebaceous glands in the skin. The resultant oily skin fosters bacterial infection. In recent years many doctors have emphasized the use of antibiotics in treating acne. While the daily use of tetracycline or other broad-spectrum antibiotics may indeed help to control the inflammation and infection of this upsetting condition, we must once again point out that the habitual use of antibiotics can have undesirable side effects, including the proliferation of resistant organisms and disturbances in the balance of intestinal bacteria, among many other results. For this reason it is wise to look for alternatives to drug treatment, and in the case of acne there is ample justification to turn to diet as the first approach.

Diet

We know that the production of sebum (the secretion of the sebaceous glands) is increased by dietary factors such as allergenic foods, overeating, excess carbohydrate and indigestible fat; moreover, digestive problems may aggravate the condition. Thus it is reasonable to expect that a carefully regulated diet would have a favorable effect.

Of course you will want to have your doctor look for possible allergies that are contributing to the condition.

Whether or not specific allergenic substances are identified, the diet should be made up of simple foods, simply prepared, such as milk, eggs, fruits, vegetables, lean meats, and liver (except when there are allergies to any of these foods). Raw fruits or vegetables should be eaten at each meal to help elimination. Certain foods sometimes aggravate acne, and such common offenders as candies, pastry, chocolate, peanut butter, sugar, colored cheeses, sodas, ketchup, French fries, hamburgers, and greasy fast foods should be eliminated from the diet, as well as highly seasoned stimulating or indigestible foods. It has also been found that bromides and iodides tend to irritate the skin, and so iodized salt, kelp, baking powder containing bromates, and other foods containing these substances should not be used.

To help enforce this dietary regimen, your child should take lunch to school and not be allowed to eat in the cafeteria. It may be necessary to make sure your youngster doesn't have extra money to spend during the school day, to prevent the purchase of harmful junk foods.

Of course, you must also be on the lookout for possible allergenic substances such as certain soaps and other cosmetics.

Herbal Preparations

It is very important to catch cases of pimples early, before aggravated eruptions occur. At the first signs of "breaking out," prepare the following *external* application:

Goldenseal. 1 teaspoonful steeped in 1 cup of boiling water. Apply to the skin, after the liquid has cooled, 2 to 3 times a day.

After applying this astringent solution to the skin, apply a *nonpenetrating* oil *lightly,* to prevent drying of the skin and to reestablish the natural balance of skin oil.

To promote proper bowel function, you may also use *senna,* as described below, for acne rosacea.

Acne rosacea, or *rosacea,* is another skin condition that may appear alone or in combination with acne vulgaris. Most common among middle-aged people, it also occurs in children and young adults. It consists of an accentuated reddening of the flush areas of the face, and there may be a skin eruption. This relatively harmless condition may be brought on by certain foods, especially stimulating and irritating substances such as spices, coffee, tea, and alcohol, as well as chocolate, nuts, and very hot or very cold foods.

Diet

A simple, bland diet of fermented dairy, fruits, vegetables, and a small serving of meat, served warm but not hot, will be helpful in this condition, with all spices, condiments, sauces, gravies, sweets, fried foods, stimulating beverages, and iodized salt and related substances discontinued. Overeating should be avoided. The bowels should be kept open, with herbal preparations if necessary. Reducing protein or carbohydrate intake will help control intestinal putrefaction and fermentation, respectively.

Herbal Preparations

To combat constipation, add *senna* leaves to fruit before cooking, and give plenty of fluids between meals. You may also make an herbal tea of *senna,* ½ teaspoon, steeped in 1 cup of freshly boiled water in a covered container for ½ hour. Drink warm or cool, 1 swallow or 1 tablespoon at a time.

ABDOMINAL PAIN. *See* COLIC

AIR SWALLOWING.
See REGURGITATION, NAUSEA, AND VOMITING

ALLERGY

Doctors often define allergy as an abnormal sensitivity to a substance that in a normal person usually produces no reaction. The substance that excites the allergic reaction is known as an "allergen." There appears to be a hereditary component in many cases of allergy, but heredity alone is not enough to produce an allergic reaction; there must also be exposure to the specific allergen to which an individual is sensitive. Different sorts of allergies predominate at different stages of childhood; among infants food allergies are most common, while in early childhood either foods or inhaled substances are the most usual allergens, and in later childhood inhalants are the main culprits. Allergic symptoms may take many forms. In the first six months of life the most common is eczema, which usually clears by the third year; asthma is the next most frequent and usually appears after the third year; hives, or urticaria, may begin after the sixth month, and many other forms of allergy begin in the later years of childhood.

When your child has an allergic reaction, your doctor will need to look for the underlying cause by taking a careful allergic history of your child and other family members. Often it is possible to date the onset of symptoms to the time when a specific food was added to the diet, but often symptoms are delayed and so this is not always a reliable guide. Your child's food dislikes are very frequently indicators of an instinctive avoidance of allergenic foods. In any infant who is bothered by skin, digestive, or neurocirculatory problems, allergy should be suspected.

Diet

Identifying Allergenic Foods. Your doctor may look for the offending food or foods in a number of possible ways. Skin-testing is one of the commonest ways of determining specific allergies. Much simpler, however, are dietary tests. The easiest test diet, known as an *empirical diet,* consists of giving your child a diet free of commonly allergenic foods (see Table 11), which are usually responsible for reactions in infants. In older children the offend-

TABLE 11
Common Allergenic Foods*

Cereals		Vegetables	
Wheat		Legumes (beans, peas, lentils)	
Wheat products		White potato	
Corn		Tomato	
Rice		Celery	
Oats		Cabbage	
Barley		Cauliflower	
Rye		Mushroom	
		Lettuce	
Dairy		Pepper	
Egg			
Milk			
Milk products		**Meats**	
		Pork	Brain
		Fish	Lung
Fruits		Beef	Chicken
Orange	Grapefruit	Lamb	Gelatin
Apple	Cantaloupe		
Banana	Grape	**Fats**	
Strawberry		Chocolate	
Peach		Nuts	

*After Kugelmass (1940).

ing food is more often an unusual one. A complete list is made of all foods eaten in the twenty-four hours prior to the allergic attack, and then your child is put on a simple diet eliminating all suspect foods on this list as well as all other commonly allergenic foods. Keeping a food diary can thus be a useful way of identifying allergenic foods in allergic children. Since processed foods generally contain a number of possible allergens, this is another very good reason to eliminate them from the diet of an allergy-prone youngster. The final diet prescribed in the empirical approach should reflect your child's likes and dislikes as well as the foods to which she is not allergic, since they must appeal to her if they are to be eaten.

The *addition diet* is another simple approach to determining food sensitivity. Your child is placed on a single food such as evaporated goat's milk with added nonallergenic sweetener, or soy milk, for three days. If no reaction occurs, then another food is added every twenty-four hours. If there is any reaction within hours after giving the new food, it is considered allergenic and eliminated from the diet. Proteins should be added first, then carbohydrates, and finally fats. Organ meats are less likely to be allergenic than muscle meats or fish. The most commonly allergenic foods should not be included among the gradual food additions.

The *elimination diet* is a more sophisticated way to determine food sensitivities. Table 12 shows three types of diet that contain generally nonallergenic foods. Your child is placed on the first diet for a week; if allergic symptoms are relieved, the foods indicated may be added gradually. If the allergic condition persists, try the second and then the third diet. If all three diets fail to bring relief, then your child will need to be maintained on soy milk with calories provided as added sweetener (blackstrap molasses or other nonallergenic sugar), starch, and oil, along with vitamin and mineral supplements, until desensitization procedures can be carried out.

Food Desensitization. Many children outgrow their food allergies, and the most effective way to desensitize

TABLE 12
Elimination Diets*

Foods	Group 1	Group 2	Group 3
Cereal	Tapioca Rice products	Corn products	Tapioca
Flour (for bread, etc.)	Rice	Corn Rye (100% rye)	Lima bean Soy Potato
Meat	Lamb Gelatin	Chicken Bacon Gelatin	Beef Bacon Gelatin
Vegetables	Spinach Lettuce Carrot Beet Artichoke	Corn Tomato Asparagus Peas String beans Squash	Lima beans Potato, white Potato, sweet Beet String beans Tomato Carrot
Fruits	Grapefruit Lemon Pears	Apricots Peaches Prunes Pineapple	Grapefruit Lemon Peaches Apricots

Additions	Cane sugar*
	Cottonseed oil*
	Olive oil
	Syrup from maple
	    sugar or cane*
		Cane sugar*
		Cottonseed oil*
		Corn oil
		Corn syrup*
		Vitamin con-
		    centrates
			Cane sugar*
			Cottonseed oil*
			Olive oil
			Syrup from maple
			    sugar or cane*

*The diets as given (after Kugelmass, 1940) reflect conventional medical practice. Under your physician's supervision, you may wish to make *cautious* substitutions for foods not generally recommended in this book.

your child to allergenic foods is to eliminate them from the diet. If this is difficult, then your doctor may choose to give your child desensitization treatment in the form of shots or of tiny, gradually increasing quantities of the offending food by mouth. Desensitizing your child to a specific food will require eliminating it from the diet for a considerable period of time; it may take months before any tolerance is achieved. The initial diet should be based on foods that have not produced allergic reactions in the past; usually a balanced diet can be formulated including some form of milk or milk substitute, with or without added sweetener; two fruits, two vegetables, meats, and unsalted butter. All foods should be cooked, and new foods should be added in small amounts to determine your child's tolerance. If an allergic reaction occurs after the addition of any food, it should be excluded from the diet.

Common Allergenic Foods. Knowing which foods most commonly produce allergic reactions in children, and how they may best be prepared to avoid reactions, will be helpful in putting together your child's desensitizing diet.

Among the most common of all food allergens is *wheat.* Other cereals may also produce allergic reactions, the most common being corn, rice, oats, barley, and rye. It seems that the cereals (and other foods also) that are most widely eaten are the ones that tend most often to produce allergic reactions.

Milk is another food to which many children are sensitive. Children may be intolerant of milk because of a true allergy to milk protein, or because they lack sufficient quantities of the enzyme lactase to digest the lactose, or milk sugar, present in milk and other dairy products. (See the separate discussion of these problems under "Milk Intolerance," beginning on page 238.)

Egg is another common allergen for children. Usually it is the egg white to which they are sensitive, but sometimes it is the yolk; and in any case it can sometimes be difficult to feed one without the other. Because egg allergy is so common, it is a good idea to introduce egg cautiously even to normal infants, giving only the yolk in tiny amounts to make sure they can tolerate it, and to exclude egg entirely from the diet of any allergy-prone infant or child. Egg allergy gradually decreases with age.

An added problem with wheat, egg, and milk is that they are used as ingredients in a nearly unlimited variety of other foods, and so it is important to know exactly what ingredients are in anything you offer an allergic child. Table 13 lists some foods that contain none of these three allergens. Avoid processed foods especially, since they are likely to contain one or more of the common offenders.*

Many children are allergic to *meat* proteins, generally developing symptoms of intestinal indigestion. The most commonly offending meat proteins are pork, beef, lamb, brain, lung, chicken, and gelatin. Less-commonly-eaten meats such as duck, goose, goat, pheasant, and venison rarely produce symptoms except sometimes in individuals who regularly eat these foods. Cooking meat greatly reduces its allergenic properties.

Fish, and especially *shellfish,* are capable of producing very violent allergic reactions; in very sensitive children even skin contact with fish, or the smell of it alone, may be enough to trigger allergic symptoms. Unlike other foods, fish doesn't lose much of its allergenic properties through cooking. Allergic children may need to eliminate fish-oil supplements from their diet, using water-soluble forms of vitamins A and D instead.

The most commonly allergenic *fruits* are oranges, apples, bananas, strawberries, and melons. Raw fruits are more usually the problem, but some children may react more strongly to cooked fruits. Among *vegetables,* the legume family is the most commonly allergenic, other frequent offenders being white potato, tomato, celery,

---

*The recipes in Book IV are all egg- and dairy-free, so you will find many of them useful in a nonallergenic diet.

TABLE 13
Milk-, Wheat-, Egg-Free Foods*

Cereals	Milk Substitutes	Fats
Cornmeal	Soy and other	Vegetable oils
Cornstarch	vegetable milks	Fish oils
Barley flour		Bacon fat
Oats, rolled	**Fruits**	Meat fats
Potato flour	Raw, stewed, or	Avocado
Soy flour	frozen (without	Nuts
Rice flour	milk or cream)	
Rye		**Sweets**
Cassava flour	**Vegetables**	Refined sugars
Corn	Raw, cooked, or	Molasses
Barley, pearled	frozen (made	Honey
Hominy	without milk,	Jams and jellies,
Sago	wheat or egg	homemade
Tapioca	products)	Corn syrup
Cream of barley		
Rice flakes	**Meats**	
Rice crispies	Any meat (pre-	
Rice, puffed	pared without	
Corn flakes	milk, wheat, or	
Cream of rye	egg products)	
Rice biscuits		

Breads
Rice bread
Ry-Krisp
Cornbread

*After Kugelmass (1940).

cabbage, cauliflower, and mushroom. Cooking will reduce the allergenic properties of vegetables, and therefore the allergic child should be maintained on cooked, nonallergenic vegetables such as spinach, beets, carrots, artichoke, turnip, and sweet potato.

Herbal Preparations

Although it is generally safe for all children and infants, *chamomile* is *to be avoided* by allergic individuals.

A safe and soothing herbal tea for allergy-prone youngsters is *passionflower,* ¼ to ½ teaspoon of the herb to 1 cup of freshly boiled water. Cover and steep for 5–10 minutes. Drink warm.

APPENDICITIS

There seems to be a strong hereditary factor in appendicitis, and so if your family has a predisposition to this disorder, it is wise to remember that diet may be a significant help in prevention.

Diet

Prevention. Two things that seem to favor the development of appendicitis are constipation and unbalanced nutrient intake; both of these can be corrected through proper diet. Meals should provide adequate calories and nutrients, but overfeeding must be avoided. Allergic children should not be given foods that tend to produce allergic reactions in the digestive system. Although the reason is not clear, children in warm climates who eat mainly fresh fruits and vegetables are remarkably free of appendicitis, and so you would do well to follow their example and make sure that your child eats plenty of fresh fruits, vegetables, and whole grains and avoids sugary and devitalized junk foods.

Acute Attack. If your child has a pain in the abdomen that persists for an hour or more, *call your doctor.* The symptoms of appendicitis vary so greatly that it is dangerous to take a chance on missing the diagnosis. When appendicitis is suspected, your child should be put in bed and given no foods except for fluids every hour, such as weak nonlaxative herb tea with added blackstrap molasses, strained fruit juice, or water with blackstrap molasses flavored with fruit juice. If vomiting is present, you may not be able to get these fluids down; vomiting may be helped by giving cracked ice, iced carbonated water, or dilute lime water every hour.

If the diagnosis is appendicitis, your doctor will probably recommend immediate surgery. If the attack subsides, however, keep your child on a liquid diet for a week—skim or acid milk, clear broth, thin cereal, gruels and strained fruit, with fruit juices given between meals. Then begin adding other foods one at a time as tolerated, avoiding any that may produce digestive-system reactions if your child is allergy-prone. If your child has a tendency to constipation, be sure to provide a diet that will help keep the bowels open (see "Constipation").

Postsurgery. If appendectomy is performed, don't take it for granted that your child will be provided with the proper foods while in the hospital. Regrettably, hospital diets are often poorly balanced and loaded with devitalized sugary and starchy foods. During the first twenty-four hours after surgery your child will receive nothing but fluids, but you may want to watch out thereafter to be sure that he is not being given allergenic foods, or overly processed or sugared meals.

Herbal Preparations

During an acute attack of suspected appendicitis, you may prepare a soothing herbal tea of any of the following (safe for infants also). These herbs are always good to use with children, and might be made a little weaker than usual at this particular time.

| *Chamomile* or *Anise* or *Fennel* | Place ½ teaspoon of selected herb in a pot. Add 1 cup freshly boiled water. Cover and steep for 5–10 minutes. Strain. Drink warm. (A *hibiscus* leaf may be added to any of these herbs for flavoring.) |

To help control constipation, a commercial herbal laxative, Swiss-Kriss, is gentle and effective for children. Use ¼ of the adult dose. Other gentle laxatives include:

Senna. ½ teaspoon of the leaves to 1 cup of freshly boiled water. Cover and steep for 5–10 minutes. Strain. Drink warm, one swallow or 1 tablespoon at a time.

Slippery elm. ½ teaspoon of the bark added to 1½ pints boiling water. Cover and continue boiling at a slow boil for about 30 minutes. Allow to cool slowly in the closed container. Drink cold, one swallow or 1 tablespoon at a time.

ASTHMA (BRONCHIAL ASTHMA)

This disorder, very common among children of all ages, is characterized by attacks of paroxysmal shortness of breath owing to blockage of the air passages in the lungs. The most common cause is allergy. In older children the allergen is most often an inhaled substance, while in very young children the offending substances are usually foods.

Treatment of an acute attack of asthma is addressed to relieving the symptoms; your pediatrician will likely prescribe medications to keep on hand for an asthmatic youngster. During an attack your child should be kept quiet, warm, and comfortable; adults must not show undue anxiety in his presence. If a suspected allergenic food has been eaten recently, it may be removed from the stomach by the use of an emetic such as ipecac syrup, or if the attack is more delayed, the bowels may be cleared by an enema. If your child can't take much fluid by mouth, your doctor may suggest artificial means of giving fluids. Your child's refusal of food and drink is actually a protective mechanism, not only to guard against allergenic foods but also because anything in the stomach may aggravate the attack.

Diet

When your child is ready to eat, he should be given foods that were well tolerated in the past, emphasizing high-carbohydrate, fat-free foods, and alkaline-forming fruits and vegetables during the attack. (See Table 16 under "Constipation," page 184.)

Breast-fed infants may develop an asthmatic attack owing to the presence of an allergen in the mother's milk. If skin-testing on your baby shows allergy to certain foods, these should be eliminated from the mother's diet throughout the nursing period, as should any foods to which your baby showed any sort of allergic reaction in the past. If no specific substances can be identified through skin-testing, the mother should eliminate commonly allergenic foods from her diet such as egg, wheat, and chocolate, limiting her milk intake to a cup of *natural* yogurt with each meal. She should also treat constipation since it might result in allergens' being absorbed from her intestinal tract and ending up in her milk. (See "Herbal Preparations" below for herbal remedies for constipation.)

During the attack, a liquid diet should first be given, consisting of dilute evaporated milk acidified with lactic acid for young infants, as well as weak herbal tea and cooked fruit juice for older children. After this preliminary period of reduced feeding, other nonallergenic foods may be added gradually, such as nonwheat cereals, noncitrus fruits, nonleguminous vegetables, and boiled meats. As much fluid as can be tolerated should be given during the acute attack to prevent dehydration and to liquefy the bronchial secretions. Even water may contain allergenic substances of animal or vegetable origin, and so it should be boiled.

Chronic asthmatic attacks are more often due to food allergy than to other causes. Chronic food allergy is usually marked by loss of appetite and digestive disturbances, and the diet should be carefully selected to fulfill all nutritional requirements to maintain health and growth. If specific foods are determined to be allergenic for your child, they should be eliminated from the diet and replaced by nonallergenic foods of equivalent food value. A diet high in fat, low in carbohydrate, and with moderate protein, with minimal amounts of salt and water, will be helpful after recovery from an acute attack. This so-called ketogenic diet (which produces ketone bodies in the urine) will somewhat dehydrate the tissues, which helps to suppress allergic reactions. Meals should be simple and well cooked, with the biggest meal at midday and a light supper of nonallergenic foods, with no eating between meals or at bedtime. Digestive disturbances may bring on an attack, so everything possible should be done to promote a well-regulated diet, normal elimination, periodic rest, and avoidance of emotional upset. A good digestive supplement, containing digestive enzymes, given before meals, may help prevent indigestion.

In formulating a preventive diet for your child, remember that it isn't enough to provide a well-balanced combination of nonallergenic foods; they must also be appealing enough so that they will actually be eaten, and so consider the palatability of meals as well as their nutritional value. Again, the final diet should be a ketogenic, dehydrating type as described above. Such a diet, free of allergenic foods, if maintained for several months, should result in improvement in the asthmatic condition and produce desensitization to the foods that brought on attacks in the past. Of course, it will also be necessary to control your child's environment, removing any inhaled or other substances that may be allergenic (house dust, for example, is a common offender). Your doctor may also advise desensitization therapy.

Herbal Preparations

Ephedra ("Mormon Tea"). The well-known over-the-counter medication Sudafed is so named for "pseudoephedrine." The "real" ephedrine is an alkaloid found in over forty species of plants, several of which have been used to treat asthmatic symptoms in China for thousands of years. This compound dilates the bronchioles and increases blood pressure.

Steep ½ teaspoonful of the herb in 2 cups of boiling water, for 5–20 minutes (steep, do not boil). Taken ½ to 1 cup daily, it has relieved the symptoms of bronchial asthma.

See "Herbal Preparations" on page 188 for gentle laxatives to keep the bowels open. Nursing mothers should take *twice* the children's dose indicated.

See also ALLERGY

BEDWETTING (ENURESIS)

There may be many different causes for bedwetting in children over five or six years of age, ranging from mechanical problems through allergic or psychological disturbances. No matter what the underlying cause, however, it will certainly help to provide your child with a diet that does not aggravate the problem. Your doctor will help to determine if there are abnormalities in the urine itself that call for medical or dietary intervention, such as excess uric acid, sugar, or ketone bodies.

Diet

In general, the preferred diet for bedwetting consists of dry, nonirritating foods, well cooked and served without spices or condiments, and with no stimulating beverages such as cocoa, coffee, tea, or caffeine-containing soft drinks. Foods that are difficult to digest, such as preserved meats, yellow cheese, and mushrooms, should also be avoided, since these will irritate the bladder. If skin tests show food allergies, eliminate these items from your child's diet. Raw foods and uncooked fruit juices should also be eliminated from the diet since they may irritate the bladder or intestines.

While it might seem reasonable to restrict fluid intake between meals, this can lead to a highly concentrated urine that will irritate the bladder. However, fluids should be restricted five hours before bedtime, and supper should be a small, dry meal relatively high in fat, which tends to reduce urinary output. Protein and carbohydrate, on the other hand, tend to increase urinary secretion. Adding salt to food at the end of the day will also help your child's body tissues to retain fluids through the night.

The basic diet, then, should consist of a normal breakfast and lunch, with most of the fluid given in the morning, less at noon, even less in the afternoon, and none after 4 P.M. Supper may consist of eggs, meat, fish, or cottage cheese, avocado and oil, or dried fruit and a little cream, bread and butter. The recommended salt may be given at supper or in a snack at bedtime, such as whole-wheat crackers with deviled ham or salty fish.

Herbal Preparations

To promote proper function of the urinary organs, give any one of the following herbs as a tea. Remember that as with all fluids, such herbal teas should be given early in the day, and never later than five hours before bedtime.

Bearberry   Place ½ teaspoon of selected herb
or *Plantain*   in a pot. Add 1 cup freshly boiled
or *Fennel*   water. Cover and steep for 5–10
                     minutes. Drink warm.

BRONCHITIS

This infection of the bronchial tubes may start as a cold and spread downward, leading to cough, rattling or squeaking noises due to mucus, and sometimes fever. The cough and noises on breathing may resemble asthma, but if there is a fever over 101° (or whatever danger point you and your doctor agree on), *call your pediatrician*. Remember that even milder fevers normally go up at night in children; but if the fever does not break overnight, or if wheezing and hacking cough persist, even if no fever is present, *consult your doctor*. He will be able to tell if there is an infection present and may choose to treat it with antibiotics.

Diet

You can continue to feed a breast-fed infant normally unless there is difficulty breathing, in which case you may need to express breast milk manually and feed it by bottle, feeder, or spoon; similar methods may have to be used with bottle-fed infants. Older children should be limited to easily digestible foods—thin cereals, strained fruit, warm skim milk—with the total amount cut in half to prevent digestive disturbances. The cough of bronchitis can be quite debilitating, and to help keep up your child's strength you may add extra calories in the form of blackstrap molasses in food or fruit juices. When the acute stage of the illness subsides, return to normal quantities of nutrients.

When bronchitis is a chronic problem, it is necessary for your doctor to look for the underlying cause and also for possible nutritional deficiencies. Sunlight, fresh air, plenty of rest and sleep, and excellent nutrition will help prevent the possible serious complications of chronic bronchitis. A prolonged episode will require a high-calorie, concentrated diet, with feedings given every four hours, and with extra vitamin and mineral supplements in addition to the usual Longevity Formula (see Appendix B), in order to preserve your child's strength. You may need to increase the amount of food gradually in order to reach the proper level of increased intake, avoiding overly bulky foods that will fill your child up before enough calories have been taken in.

Herbal Preparations

Herbal Vaporizer Mix. Use vaporizer at night to relieve congestion. The herbal mix consists of ½ ounce each of *boneset, burdock,* and *eucalyptus.* Place herbs in a cheesecloth bag and boil for 20 minutes in 2 quarts of water. Strain. Place liquid in vaporizer, then dilute with water to reach proper level.

Acacia Gum. Suck on dried gum to soothe bronchial passages.

The following herbs, used singly, make soothing teas:

Eucalyptus
or *Grindelia*
or *Horehound*
or *Wild-cherry bark*
or *Yerba santa*

Place ½ teaspoon of selected herb in a pot. Add 1 cup of freshly boiled water. Cover and steep for 5–10 minutes. Drink warm.

Licorice
or *Pleurisy Root*

Add ½ teaspoon of selected herb to 1½ pints boiling water. Cover and continue boiling at a slow boil for about 30 minutes. Allow to cool slowly in the closed container. Drink cold, one swallow or one tablespoon at a time.

CELIAC DISEASE

This malabsorption syndrome may first appear at age 6–18 months, and is marked by loose, frequent, foul-smelling stools, sometimes with intermittent constipation. The child appears miserable and wasted, with poor appetite and distended abdomen. The cause has been determined to be an inability of the system to digest gluten, a protein substance found in wheat, as well as all other grains except rice and corn.

Diet

The treatment of celiac disease is through a diet that eliminates all wheat, rye, oats, barley, and buckwheat, and any products made from them. Since these grains are used in an extremely wide variety of processed and packaged foods, it is imperative that you become expert at reading labels to determine whether the foods you buy contain any of these grains or their derivatives. Flour and cereal products are also used in preparing gravies, sauces, and many other foods, and so you must also be aware of how dishes are made so that you can guard against these grain products when you are eating dinner at a restaurant or at a friend's home.

Your pediatrician will advise you on how to provide adequate, balanced nutrition for your child while avoiding the prohibited foods. Table 14 lists some of the foods permitted and to be avoided on the gluten-free diet.

Herbal Preparations

Soothing herbal teas may be made of any of the following:

Goldenseal. Add ½ teaspoon of the root to 1 pint of boiling water. Cover and continue boiling at a slow boil for about 30 minutes. Allow to cool slowly in the closed container. Drink cold, one swallow or 1 tablespoon at a time.

or *Balm of Gilead* or *Mullein*	Place ½ teaspoon of selected herb in a pot. Add 1 cup freshly boiled water. Cover and steep for 5–10 minutes. Drink cold, one swallow or 1 tablespoon at a time.

COLDS

The common cold is a viral infection that may take a number of different forms. Fever may or may not be present, as may loss of appetite, nausea and vomiting, and nasal stuffiness. All these factors can influence your child's ability and desire to eat. In order to protect against superimposed bacterial infections during this period of lowered resistance, it is important to maintain as good nutrition as possible and to encourage plenty of fluid intake. Until you are familiar with the particular pattern that colds follow in your child, it is a good idea to *consult your doctor* when cold symptoms appear, and *always* when there is a very high fever or any deviation from the course of events you have come to expect. The vitamin-C "cocktail" described on page 147 should be given in addition to the usual supplement formula.

Diet

Infants should be continued on breast- or bottle-feedings, with plenty of water or fruit juice with added blackstrap molasses between feedings, other foods being discontinued. To reduce the risk of digestive problems and vomiting, limit feedings to the amount your child can tolerate; breast-fed infants may need to have their

TABLE 14
Gluten-Free Diet*

Type of Food	Foods Allowed	Foods Excluded
Beverages	Mineral water, herb tea, wine	Cereal beverages, cocoa mixes, malted drinks, nondairy creamers, ale, beer, many distilled liquors made from excluded grains
Milk and Dairy	Whole, dry, or fermented milk, cream, sour cream, yogurt. Natural, aged cheeses, cottage cheese (check vegetable gum used)	Malted milk Cheese spreads; any cheese product containing oat gum
Meat, fish, poultry	All fresh meats, fish, shellfish, poultry; fish canned in oil or brine; prepared meat products which don't contain prohibited ingredients	Processed meats containing wheat, rye, oats, or barley, such as some sausages, hot dogs, luncheon meats, etc; meat dishes containing bread or bread crumbs (meat loaf, croquettes); some tuna canned in vegetable broth; bread stuffings; gravies thickened with flour
Eggs	Plain eggs, or eggs used in cooking	Eggs in sauces made of gluten-containing ingredients
Bread	Bread or muffins made with arrowroot, potato, rice, corn, or soy flour	Any bread products made with wheat, rye, barley, or oat flour; pretzels, crackers, pancakes, mixes

[174]

Type of Food	Foods Allowed	Foods Excluded
Cereal	Rice and corn cereals; cornmeal, hominy, rice	Any cereal made with oats, wheat, rye, bran, malt, barley, buckwheat; pasta
Vegetables	All plain, fresh, frozen or canned vegetables; dried peas, beans, lentils; potatoes	Any commercially prepared vegetables made with gluten-containing ingredients; creamed vegetables; canned baked beans; commercially prepared salads
Soups	Homemade broth; bouillon; vegetable and cream soups thickened with cornstarch or potato flour only	Any soups containing prohibited flours or starches
Fruits	All plain fruits and juices	Thickened or prepared fruits; some pie fillings
Desserts and Sweets	Custards, puddings, blancmange made from allowable flours and starches; gelatin desserts; sherbet; tapioca; homemade ice cream; homemade jams and jellies; honey; molasses	Baked goods containing wheat, rye, barley, or oat products, such as cakes, cookies, ice cream, pastries, pies, puddings, or desserts made from commercial mixes
Miscellaneous	Salt, spices, herbs, pickles, vinegar, nuts, olives, peanut butter	Gravies or sauces thickened with prohibited flours; bottled meat sauces; malt extract; flavoring syrups

*This diet has been adapted from several sources and reflects the general dietary recommendations made in this book, omitting such items as refined sugars and carbonated drinks from the list of permitted foods. Some foods, such as wine, may not be suitable for children but are listed for your information.

nursing periods shortened. Bottle-fed infants may have their feedings thickened with barley flour, with the amount reduced to half of normal. If your infant has trouble taking adequate fluid, your doctor may choose to give additional fluids by artificial means.

Sugar in formulas may produce diarrhea, in which case a little blackstrap molasses may be substituted, with a little grated raw apple pulp given between feedings to help control the diarrhea. Digestive problems associated with fever will clear up as the temperature returns to normal, and as appetite improves, foods can be added gradually until the diet is back to normal.

In older children, a soft diet should be given during fever (see Table 23, page 209), with hourly water and fruit juices with blackstrap molasses. Reducing food intake generally protects against digestive troubles; of course, any foods known to produce allergic digestive disturbances should be avoided. All foods should be cooked, strained, and given in small, frequent feedings. If there is nausea and vomiting, food may be withheld for twelve hours, or limited to skim milk; your doctor may recommend additional fluids to be administered artificially. Diarrhea may be relieved by giving only boiled skim milk and banana, with raw grated apple pulp between feedings. As temperature subsides, your child's appetite will return, and she can resume a normal, balanced diet.

Herbal Preparations

To help break up the symptoms of a cold, make a tea of one of the following herbs:

Boneset	Place ½ teaspoon of selected herb
or *Ginger*	in a pot. Add 1 cup freshly boiled
or *Yerba Santa*	water. Cover and steep for 5–10
	minutes. Drink warm.

COLIC

The spasmodic abdominal pains known as colic may be a sign of digestive problems or other disorders. The immediate cause of these pains may be overdistension of the stomach and intestines with gas, or forceful peristaltic contractions of the digestive tract, or a combination of these factors. The paroxysmal nature of the pains distinguishes colic from the steadier abdominal pain of inflammations or other disorders. *Your doctor must be consulted immediately* if blood appears in the urine or stool; of course, you as a parent with good common sense would do so!

Diet

Babies vary greatly in the degree to which they are bothered by colicky sensations. While colic can often be traced to an overly sensitive nervous temperament, it is always wise to look into possible dietary factors when your child shows signs of colicky pain. The accumulation of gas can be caused, for example, by excessive air swallowing in breast- or bottle-fed infants. This may happen because your baby is gulping her feedings, or perhaps because she is not receiving enough food and is experiencing painful hunger contractions or is swallowing air to compensate for the not-full feeling. Unbalanced feedings, especially excessive quantities of fat or of easily fermentable carbohydrate, are another possible cause. Breast-fed babies may be intolerant of breast milk because of a substance in the mother's diet to which they are sensitive or because they are receiving too much fat in the last portions of the milk. Strategies for dealing with these possible dietary problems may be found under the discussion of "Indigestion" (chronic intestinal). Table 24, page 211, lists foods that tend to discourage or encourage the formation of gas in the bowel.

Herbal Preparations

Any one of the following herbs may be used to prepare a gently soothing herbal tea for children of all ages, including infants:

Chamomile   Place ½ teaspoon of selected herb
or *Anise*   in a pot. Add 1 cup freshly boiled
or *Fennel*   water. Cover and steep for 5–10
                     minutes. Drink warm. (A *hibiscus*
                     leaf may be added to any of these
                     herbs for flavoring.)

COLITIS (CHRONIC ULCERATIVE)

This is an inflammatory and ulcerative disorder of the colon, characterized by the gradual onset of bloody diarrhea, which might be mistaken for dysentery. The diarrhea becomes progressively severe, blood and mucus being passed with or without stools. If you observe these symptoms, consult your physician. Since prolonged colitis can interfere with the absorption of protein and the assimilation of vitamins and minerals, deficiency states can result. The disorder tends to resolve itself spontaneously, and your doctor will prescribe a treatment program that should be supplemented with an appropriate diet.

Diet

The diet must be adjusted to your child's individual needs, but will generally be high in calories and in protein, with high vitamin and mineral content, but low in carbohydrates and in residue (see Table 15). Changes in diet will not necessarily affect the nature of the stools. In order to protect the mucous membranes of the intestines, your doctor may recommend extra vitamin and

TABLE 15
Low-Residue Foods

Cereals and Breads
Refined cereals, cooked
Arrowroot products
Crackers
Enriched white bread
Spaghetti, pasta

Soups
Strained vegetable soups
Bouillon
Broths
Cream soups

Dairy
Butter
Cottage cheese
Cream cheese
Milk
Eggs

Meats and Fish
Lean beef, lamb, chicken
Fish

Sweets
Custard
Ice cream
Gelatin

Fruits
Cooked fruits, strained or
  pureed
Fruit juices

Pudding
Honey
Molasses

Vegetables
Cooked vegetables, strained
  or pureed
Vegetable juices
Potato

Avoid
Raw fruits and vegetables
Whole-grain cereals and breads;
  bran, corn, dried legumes
Fried foods; excess fat; nuts
Pork
Highly seasoned foods
Marmalades and jams

mineral supplementation in addition to the usual supplement formula.

Herbal Preparations

To help control diarrhea without irritating the bowel, use either of the following herbs:

Spanish Chestnut: Add ½ teaspoon of leaves and bark
to 1½ pints boiling water. Cover
and continue boiling at a slow boil
for about 30 minutes. Allow to cool
slowly in the closed container. Drink
cold, one swallow or 1 tablespoon at
a time.

or *Red Raspberry:*   Place ½ teaspoon of the *leaf* in a
pot. Add 1 cup freshly boiled water.
Cover and steep for 5–10 minutes.
Drink warm. If *root bark* is used,
add ½ teaspoon to 1½ pints of boiling water. Cover and continue boiling at slow boil for about 30 minutes.
Allow to cool slowly in the closed
container. Drink cold, one swallow
or 1 tablespoon at a time.

CONSTIPATION

Constipation has been identified as a contributing
factor in many diseases owing to the retention of waste
products in the system. The term actually includes a very
complex set of symptoms, and it is important to understand what actually constitutes constipation so that you
don't become overly concerned when your child doesn't
have a bowel movement right on schedule every day.
Constipation has nothing to do with the frequency of
stools; rather, it is a symptom that indicates that fecal material is remaining too long in the intestines. As a result,

the moisture is absorbed through the walls of the intestines and the fecal mass becomes hard and dry. The result may be infrequent, sometimes painful bowel movements, and a vicious cycle can develop in which your child is afraid to pass stools because of the discomfort involved. Parental attitude can have a tremendous influence on this problem. It is very important to avoid expressing anxiety about "BMs" in the presence of your child; such anxiety is all too contagious, and may make matters worse. If you think that your child is indeed having problems with constipation, *consult your pediatrician.* There are so many possible causes that expert medical help is required.

Diet

In most cases, food is the best medicine for constipation. A balanced diet of natural, wholesome foods, such as we have advocated throughout this book, including whole grains, fresh fruits and vegetables, with appropriate amounts of dairy and meat products, and avoiding overly processed foods such as white sugar and flour, will establish a good foundation for normal bowel habits in your child. Natural, dietary treatment of constipation is vastly preferable to the use of enemas, laxatives, and other drugs, which have a psychological as well as a physical impact on your child. Unless your doctor feels such measures are called for, look for the proper dietary solution rather than artificial means for treating constipation.

In evaluating the possible causes of constipation, you will need to consider the possibility of various sorts of dietary imbalances. *Insufficient food* is one possibility. Breast-fed infants who are not receiving enough milk generally develop small diarrheal movements as the first sign of undernutrition. However, since breast milk is very completely utilized by your baby's body, it leaves little or no residue, and if he is not getting enough milk, constipation may result. Increasing the amount of food will clear the constipation in such cases. *Your pediatri-*

cian must be consulted in any case where your baby is not receiving enough milk; if the supply of breast milk can't be increased, he may recommend supplementary bottle-feedings. Meanwhile, the mother should review her own diet and try to improve her nutritional status in an effort to increase the quantity of her milk. Bottle-fed infants, similarly, may have so little residue from insufficient amounts of food, or from highly diluted feedings, that there is not enough residue to stimulate elimination. Again, increasing the nutrient content of the feeding and perhaps using more concentrated feedings should solve the problem. Older children may also become constipated because of inadequate or too completely absorbed foods, usually owing to their refusing foods or receiving too limited a diet. If you suspect that this is the reason for constipation in your child, increase the total food intake, especially of residue-producing foods such as whole-grain bread, bran biscuits, raw and dried fruits, green vegetables, butter and cream. If these are the sorts of foods your child resists, combine them with things he likes better.

Insufficient fluid intake is another common cause of constipation. Especially during the warm summer months, a breast-fed infant may produce overly well formed stools that contain little fluid. Orange juice won't help much unless given in very large amounts, but prune, fig, date, or apricot juice will be a very effective addition to your baby's fluid intake because these juices contain natural sugars that have laxative properties. Bottle-fed infants who are receiving concentrated-milk mixtures will need to have their fluid intake increased between feedings, with fruit juices, especially prune juice, or blackstrap molasses diluted in water, given before regular feedings. Older children may also get into the habit of not taking enough fluids. Make sure your child is drinking plenty of water during the day, and give him lots of fruit juice, beginning when he first gets up in the morning and on a regular schedule throughout the day. Unless he drinks at least three glasses of fluids a day, his stool will tend to get dried out.

Protein-Carbohydrate Imbalance. Foods high in protein are known as *acid-forming,* and tend to produce constipation, while those high in carbohydrates are *alkaline-forming,* and tend to have a laxative effect. The acid- or alkali-forming properties of foods are due to the mineral residue that remains after the combustible portion of the food has been "burned" in the body. Eggs, meat, and cereal are the most acid-forming foods, while fruits, vegetables, and milk are the best alkaline-forming foods. It may seem paradoxical that acid-tasting fruits form alkalis in the body, but the minerals they leave behind after being burned as fuel are in fact alkaline. It is particularly important for children to eat large quantities of alkaline-forming foods, since the alkaline minerals are involved in the binding of protein in tissue formation. Table 16 lists some common foods that are acid- and alkaline-forming, and some that are neutral in this regard.

Protein-carbohydrate imbalance is not usually a problem in breast-fed babies, since human milk contains these nutrients in the ideal proportions for proper utilization and elimination. Bottle-fed infants, however, may develop constipation if they are being given large amounts of milk with little added carbohydrate. Sugar has a naturally laxative effect, and so increasing the content of sweetener in the formula will help with this problem. Adding blackstrap molasses or other sweetener to the formula, *under your pediatrician's supervision,* may be helpful in correcting constipation. Older children may also be receiving a diet disproportionately high in protein and low in carbohydrate. The natural sugars in dried and fresh fruits, as well as whole-grain bread, coarse cereals such as oatmeal, cornmeal, cracked wheat and bran, and blackstrap molasses are useful dietary additions. It will also help to change the protein content from muscle meats to organ meats (liver, brains, etc.), and to increase butter, cream, and oil intake, as well as fresh fruits and vegetables.

Excessive fat can also produce constipation. In breast-fed infants this may occur when they nurse for

TABLE 16
Acid- and Alkali-Forming Foods*

High-Acid Foods (in decreasing order of acid content)	High-Alkali Foods (in decreasing order of alkali content)
Bread and Cereals	**Dairy**
Whole wheat	Milk, fermented
Shredded wheat	Milk, whole
Barley	Milk, skim
Rice	
Corn flakes	**Fruits**
Crackers	Figs, dried
Whole-wheat bread	Bananas
White bread	Pineapple
	Apricots, dried
Dairy	Watermelon
Egg yolk	Peaches
Whole egg	Cantaloupe
Egg white	Strawberries
American cheese	Oranges
	Apples
Fish	Pears
Mackerel	Coconut
Cod	
Haddock	**Nuts**
Flounder	Almonds
Halibut	Chestnuts
Whitefish	
Salmon	**Vegetables**
Oysters	Beet greens
Smelt	Carrots
Trout	Spinach
	Beans, lima
Meats	Beans, string
Chicken	Brussels sprouts
Beef, lean	Turnips

High-Acid Foods (in decreasing order of acid content)	High-Alkali Foods (in decreasing order of alkali content)
Lamb chops	Potatoes, white
Corned beef, canned	Beets
Turkey	Tomatoes
Veal	Rhubarb
Ham	Lettuce
Bacon	Celery
	Peas
Vegetables and Nuts	
Walnuts	
Peanuts	
Sweet corn	

Neutral Foods					
Cream	Butter	Lard	Cornstarch	Tapioca	Sugar

*After Kugelmass (1940).

prolonged periods and receive the fat-rich last portions of the breast milk. Reduce the nursing period, offering only one breast at a feeding, and give several ounces of boiled water before the feeding to discourage excessive milk intake. Bottle-fed infants may be receiving a formula high in fat content and relatively low in sugar; changing to a lower-fat milk and increasing the added carbohydrate, in the form of blackstrap molasses or other sugars recommended by your doctor, will help. Older children who are receiving a high-fat diet also tend to be constipated, and will need to be switched to more balanced nutrient intake. Milk should be limited to a glass at each meal, warm but not boiled, with added blackstrap molasses if your pediatrician agrees. Again, the addition of whole grains, coarse cereals, fresh fruits, and green vegetables is called for.

Vitamin and mineral deficiencies, specifically of vitamins B_1 and D, calcium, and potassium, can also cause constipation owing to a reduction in the tone of the intestinal musculature. Your doctor may recommend extra supplementation if this is suspected to be a contributing factor. (Also, see Tables 10 and 12, pages 146 and 159, for foods high in these nutrients.)

Not enough roughage, or fiber, in the diet is a very common cause of constipation. Fiber, a complex substance including cellulose, is not broken down by digestive enzymes, and so it passes through the intestinal tract, providing bulk in the stool and stimulating peristaltic contractions through its irritant effect. How much fiber should be given in the diet depends on the type of constipation your child is suffering from, and so before discussing the role of fiber in your child's diet, we will need to distinguish between the two types of constipation: atonic and spastic.

Atonic Constipation. This is a symptom of weakness or reduced activity of the musculature of the intestine, and may be the result of deficiencies of vitamins B_1 or D, or of calcium or potassium salts. Other possible causes are lack of exercise, convalescence from disease, or the frequent use of enemas or medicines to produce bowel movements. The stools may be of normal consistency, but more commonly they are hard and dry because of their delayed travel through the intestine. For atonic constipation, *increase* the amount of fiber in the diet by giving more dried fruits, leafy and fibrous vegetables, and coarse breads and cereals, in order to stimulate peristalsis.

Spastic Constipation. A symptom of an overly active state of the intestinal musculature, this can result from nervous tension, habitual use of cathartic medicines to increase the bulk of stools, too much roughage in the diet, or certain diseases. Stools consist of hard, dry little balls of fecal matter that have been "pinched off" by the overly active bowel. In spastic constipation you will need to give your child a bland, nonirritating diet, *low in residue*, in order to prevent aggravation of the condition. Fruits and vegetables should be cooked and put through a sieve to remove all traces of fiber. Your doctor will help you to determine the proper diet for your child's constipation. Tables 17 and 18 list foods that will be helpful in atonic or spastic constipation, respectively, and Table 19 lists foods high and low in fiber or cellulose content.

TABLE 17
Foods Helpful in Atonic Constipation*

Dairy	Vegetables	Cereals and Breads
Sour milk	Beet greens	Oatmeal
Yogurt, kefir	Spinach	Puffed wheat
Milk, unboiled	Cabbage	Shredded wheat
	Cauliflower	Cracked wheat
Sugars	Celery	Bran, rye
Honey	Cucumber	Bran, whole wheat
Molasses	Lettuce	Oatmeal crackers
	Sprouts	Graham crackers
Fruits	String beans	Graham mush
Fig juice	Vegetables,	Cornbread
Date juice	strained	Bran bread
Prune juice		Brown bread
Figs, stewed	**Fluids**	Wild rice
Prunes, stewed	Carrot water	
Peaches	Spinach water	
Apricots	Soups:	
Apple, baked	Soya bean	
Apple, scraped	Vegetable	
Applesauce	Black bean	

*After Kugelmass (1940).

TABLE 18
Foods Helpful in Spastic Constipation*

Dairy	Meats	Fruits
Acidophilus milk	Beef, scraped	Cooked:
Fresh milk	Lamb	Prunes
Cottage cheese	Bacon	Apricots
Soft cream cheese	Chicken	Peaches
Eggs	Liver	Apples
	Sweetbreads	Pears
Cereals and Breads	Fish	Bananas
Cream of wheat	Oysters	Raw:
Oatmeal		Ripe pear
Farina	**Vegetables**	Ripe banana
Puffed rice	Tender lettuce	Orange juice
Puffed wheat	Spinach	
Rice flakes	Beets	**Desserts**
Corn flakes	Carrots	Puddings:
White rice	Peas	Rice
	String beans	Tapioca
	Squash	Prune whip
	Asparagus	Ices
	Cauliflower	Ice cream
	Tomatoes, strained	Gelatin (no artificial
	Potatoes	color or flavor)

*After Kugelmass (1940).

Herbal Preparations

A commercial herbal laxative known as Swiss-Kriss is gentle and effective for children. Use ¼ of the adult dose. Other gentle laxatives include:

Senna. ½ teaspoon of the leaves to 1 cup of freshly boiled water. Cover and steep for 5–10 minutes. Drink warm, one swallow or 1 tablespoon at a time.

TABLE 19
Cellulose Content of Foods*

High Cellulose Content		Low Cellulose Content	
Fruits	**Cereals**	**Cereals and Breads**	
Dates	Whole grains	Cereals, strained	
Figs	Bran	Gruels	
Prunes		Arrowroot products	
Raisins	**Nuts**	Crackers	
Plums	All	Bread, white	
Peaches			
Grapes		**Dairy**	
Berries		Milk	
Apples		Cream	
Bananas		Butter	
Pears		Cheese	
Pomegranates		Mayonnaise	
Melons		Eggs	
Vegetables		**Meats and Fish**	
Leafy vegetables		Chicken	
Spinach		Bacon	
Cauliflower		Meats	
Celery		Beef juice	
Corn		Fish	
Carrots		Shellfish	
Beans			
Beets		**Vegetables**	
Horseradish		Vegetable juices	
Parsnips		Soups, strained	
Peas		Purees	
Peppers, green		Vegetables, strained	
Rhubarb		Dandelion greens	
Radishes			
Pumpkin		**Fruits**	**Sweets**
Squash		Oranges	Ice cream
Sweet potatoes		Grapefruit	Cakes
Yams		Cherries	Gelatin
Turnips		Fruits, pureed	Honey
Kohlrabi		Fruit juices	Molasses
Eggplant			Sugars
Asparagus		**Fats**	Starches
Okra		Oils	
Onions			
Mushrooms			
Lentils			

*After Kugelmass (1940).

[189]

Slippery Elm. ½ teaspoon of the bark added to 1½ pints boiling water. Cover and continue boiling at a slow boil for about 30 minutes. Allow to cool slowly in the closed container. Drink cold, one swallow or 1 tablespoon at a time.

COUGH:
See Herbal Remedies under BRONCHITIS

CROUP (Chronic Obstructive Laryngitis)

Characterized by hoarseness, a spasmodic barking cough, and shortness of breath, this disorder may come on suddenly, often at night. More severe cases may be marked by fever and convulsions. Because of the threat to your child's ability to breathe, *your doctor should be called immediately.* He may recommend treatment with moist air from a vaporizer; if none is available, you can fill your bathroom with steam by running hot water. Your doctor may also remove obstructive mucus with a suction device. Clearing the breathing passages will also help improve your child's desire to eat. Remember that in emergencies, breathing problems can be treated by your fire department's rescue squad, who can administer oxygen.

Diet

The shortness of breath can be very exhausting, and so it is important to maintain your child's strength through adequate nutrition, giving a liquid diet to the upper limits of tolerance (see Table 22, page 208). Warm fluids may be most helpful. Your doctor may give additional fluids artificially if necessary.

Herbal Preparations

Herbal Vaporizer Mix. Use vaporizer at night to relieve congestion. The herbal mix consists of ½ ounce each of *boneset, burdock,* and *eucalyptus.* Place herbs in a cheesecloth bag and boil for 20 minutes in 2 quarts of water. Strain. Place in vaporizer, then dilute with water to reach proper level. Let steam all night near child.

DIABETES

"Juvenile diabetes" and "maturity-onset diabetes" are terms that have been abandoned by experts in the field of diabetes. This is so because both of these varieties of diabetes can and do occur at any age. The new standard for diagnosis of diabetes in children is a random plasma-glucose level in excess of 200 mg/dl.* A new international standard dose of glucose is now given for the oral glucose-tolerance test. The glucose dose for children is 1.75 gm/kg† body weight, the total dose not to exceed 75 grams. The new diagnostic criteria for adults show that the symptoms and complications associated with diabetes mellitus usually appear only in people who have plasma-glucose levels greater than 140 mg/dl after fasting, or who show an elevated level of plasma glucose, above 200 mg/dl, both at 1 and 2 hours after an oral glucose-tolerance test. The dose of glucose that is now used internationally to test for these levels in adults is 75 grams of glucose, in nonpregnant adults. For those interested in further details of the new diagnostic criteria for diabetes, this work appears in the journal *Diabetes,* Vol. 28, p. 1039 (1979).

Diet

It has long been thought that an excess of sugar in the urine, which is indicative of diabetes, is caused by a faulty carbohydrate metabolism. Yet careful studies have not turned up any evidence to show that excess carbohydrate intake either causes diabetes or is responsible for a

*The abbreviation "dl" is for "deciliter."
†"Kg" is for "kilogram."

poor control of the disease. Current thinking in managing this disorder through diet consists of eliminating all refined sugars, reducing fat to a great extent, greatly reducing calories, and greatly increasing the amount of unrefined carbohydrates that are eaten. (Patients with a non-insulin-dependent adult diabetes who follow such a diet, high in complex carbohydrates and low in saturated fats, cholesterol, and calories, will not only benefit from a control of this disorder but will also experience a reduction in cholesterol level.) Interestingly, in Asia, diabetics usually eat high-carbohydrate diets, up to 70 percent, and there diabetes is generally quite mild, while the incidence of coronary atherosclerosis is low.

Diabetes often begins in the uterus, when the mother swallows sugar-rich foods. Not so surprisingly, babies love sweets, even before they are born. Their sweet tooth is developed long before the actual equipment appears. If a sweetener is injected into the bloodstream of a mother, a fetus will actually begin to make swallowing motions! No other food or food compound will promote such a response. This instinctual craving for sweets is a reflection of the infant's desire for sweet breast milk; yet it is quite easy to subvert this normal desire for lactose, the sugar that is found in mother's milk. If given artificial sugar-sweetened formulas, babies will eventually reject breast milk altogether, owing to the higher degree of sweetness of the formulas.

Fructose, a simple sugar, is increasingly appearing in health foods as a substitute for the more expensive honey, or for molasses. This is a great misfortune, because although fructose does not cause as great a rise in blood-glucose concentration as does sucrose or glucose, it unfortunately can increase serum triglycerides, just as the other simple sugars can. Moreover, diabetics, who know better than to consume simple sugars such as sucrose and glucose, owing to the fact that these sugars rapidly increase the secretion of insulin, may be misled into thinking that fructose is somehow healthier for them. Unfortunately, this is not so. Fructose does have a less dramatic effect on insulin secretion, but in fact it still requires some insulin to be metabolized.

A more interesting line of treatment, from a nutritional point of view, consists of the utilization of chromium. The "glucose-tolerance factor" is composed of chromium, manganese, and zinc. Individuals who have consistently low levels of these three trace minerals also often exhibit diabetes mellitus. Now, it is noteworthy that as we get older, the levels of chromium in our tissues decline, just as they decline in diabetic patients. The therapeutic application of chromium for some non-insulin-dependent diabetic patients has improved the utilization of glucose. A study of this was done at UCLA by Drs. Rabinowitz, Levin, and Gonick, and is reported in *Metabolism*, Vol. 29, p. 355 (1980). Just as some of the more sophisticated health-food publications have been reporting, an association between chromium and carbohydrate metabolism was shown. Some adult diabetics who have used daily about 3 tablespoons of brewer's yeast, which contains chromium, have been able to reduce their requirements for insulin. Children would of course require a lesser amount, as determined in conjunction with their physician, depending on their body weight.

As a final note, please bear in mind that physical exercise has been shown to improve glucose tolerance greatly and decrease the requirement for insulin in patients with diabetes. This was reported in the *New England Journal of Medicine*, Vol. 302, p. 886 (1980).

Thus, the best approach for managing diabetes may be a combination of regular physical exercise and a high-unrefined-carbohydrate, high-fiber diet that is also concomitantly low in saturated fats, cholesterol, and calories. *Consult your doctor.*

Herbal Preparations

Israeli experiments have shown that the sulfurous component of *onion* lowers blood sugar while raising levels of insulin in the cells. We therefore highly recommend the eating of this healthful bulb—raw, boiled, or baked.

A beneficial herbal tea may be made of *nettle,* using ½ teaspoon of the granulated leaves or root to 1 cup of boiling water. Cover and steep 5–10 minutes. Drink cold, 1 tablespoon at a time.

Dandelion is another helpful herb for diabetes. Use ½ teaspoon of the *leaves,* steeped in one cup of freshly boiled water. Or, if the *root* is used, use ½ teaspoon to 1½ pints of boiling water; cover and continue boiling slowly for about 30 minutes. Cool in closed container and drink cold.

Burdock root may be prepared in the same manner as dandelion root, but be sure to use roots that are at least *one year old.*

DIARRHEA

Frequent, mushy, or watery stools, lacking their usual form, are a common symptom in many diseases, and your *doctor will help to identify the cause.* Acute cases of diarrhea may be due to infection, or they may be caused by indigestion, with any of the nutrients capable of producing the disorder. If you examine the stools carefully, you may be able to detect the offending nutrient; for example, a putrid smell indicates protein putrefaction, while a sour smell suggests the fermentation of carbohydrates.

Diet

Among the dietary causes of diarrhea is *underfeeding.* If a breast-fed infant is not receiving enough milk, the stools will become frequent and greenish. If underfeeding is suspected, *consult your pediatrician immediately* to prevent possible malnutrition in your infant. Under your doctor's supervision, some of the following dietary suggestions may prove helpful. If the breast milk can't be increased, then you will need to give complementary feedings of evaporated milk with blackstrap molasses. Bottle-fed infants whose diarrheal stools contain little food material should have their formulas reevaluated; if they are failing to grow properly, they should receive concentrated feedings of evaporated or acid milk with blackstrap molasses, with other nutrients added to make up requirements as tolerance develops.

Overfeeding may also cause diarrhea, especially in warm weather when your child's digestive capacity is reduced. Breast-fed infants simply need to have their feeding decreased in duration; bottle-fed infants may need to have their formula adjusted to reflect actual caloric requirements, with other foods withheld until the diarrhea has cleared. Fluid may be made up in the form of arrowroot, barley, or rice water, perhaps with added blackstrap molasses, between feedings. Older children may also develop diarrhea from overfeeding. If your child develops sudden diarrhea after a party, for example, try a twelve-hour period with nothing but fluids such as barley or rice water, then give boiled skim milk, adding other foods gradually as tolerated.

Bottle-fed infants may develop diarrhea because of protein-curd formation from *cow's milk,* with alkaline, offensive-smelling stools containing large, amber beanlike curds. In such cases a switch to dried, evaporated, or acidified milk will help. Allergy to the protein in cow's milk is another possible cause; switching to evaporated cow's milk, goat's or soy milk should clear up the diarrhea. Older children also may develop diarrhea from *protein intolerance,* with loose, offensive-smelling stools containing undigested meat fiber. After 12–24 hours of nothing but fluids, protein intake should be limited to small amounts of plain gelatin (no artificial coloring or flavoring!), or organ meats such as calves' brain or lung, introduced one at a time to determine tolerance. Eventually you may be able to identify the offending protein food and eliminate it from your child's diet.

A bottle-fed infant who develops frothy acid stools may be receiving *excessive carbohydrate;* a formula too high in sugars is usually the culprit. After a twelve-hour period of nothing but liquids such as arrowroot, barley, or rice water, try a mixture of boiled skim milk or lactic-acid milk with a little blackstrap molasses, in half the usual amount, given every four hours, and increasing the quantity gradually as tolerated. Older children may also develop fermentative diarrhea with loose, frothy, sour stools, produced by excessive carbohydrate, or by concentrated sugar, which tends to cause diarrhea. After twelve hours of nothing but fluids by mouth, mild cases

TABLE 20
Foods Helpful in Diarrhea*

Cereals and Breads
Cornstarch
Arrowroot
Tapioca
Rice
Barley
Wheat
Gruels
Puddings
Crackers
Toast

Fruits and Vegetables
Banana, raw
Apple, raw
Pear
Potato, white (boiled or baked, no butter)

Protein Foods
Gelatin (no artificial colors or flavors)
Chicken (without skin)
Beef (well cooked)
Eggs (poached, boiled; not fried)
Fish (broiled, baked)

Fluids
Milks:
  Skim
  Lactic acid
  Yogurt or kefir
  Whey
Broth
Milk soups
Cream soups
Strained soups
Herb teas (see listing)

*Ater Kugelmass (1940).

will generally respond to feedings of banana, raw apple, junket (natural ingredients only!), and pot cheese, with no sweets given until recovery is complete.

Excessive fat can also produce diarrhea. In breast-fed infants gray or soapy stools may be caused by the intake of excess fat from the last portions of breast milk. This problem, which is especially common in warm weather, can be resolved by cutting down the time of nursing and increasing the intervals between feedings, giving water sweetened with blackstrap molasses between feedings. A bottle-fed infant may similarly develop diarrhea from cow's milk rich in cream, from cod-liver oil, egg yolk, or other fatty foods, especially when the formula also contains fermentable carbohydrate. Switch to a skim-milk formula, introducing fatty foods cautiously according to tolerance. Older children intolerant to fat will have bulky, white, frothy, offensive-smelling stools, often aggravated by warm weather. Such fatty diarrhea should clear up with restriction of fat in the diet until tolerance is reestablished.

Table 20 lists some foods that will help in diarrhea.

Herbal Preparations

Any one of the following herbs may be used to prepare a tea that will help in diarrhea:

Red Raspberry (leaf) or *Wintergreen*	Place ½ teaspoon of selected herb in a pot. Add 1 cup freshly boiled water. Cover and steep for 5–10 minutes. Drink warm.
or *Barberry* or *Licorice* or *Madder* or *Pomegranate* or *Red raspberry* (root bark) or *Sumac* berries	Add ½ teaspoon of selected herb to 1½ pints boiling water. Cover and continue boiling at a slow boil for about 30 minutes. Allow to cool slowly in the closed container. Drink cold, one swallow or 1 tablespoon at a time.

DYSENTERY

This bacterial infection of the bowel is characterized by marked diarrhea with mucus and blood in the stools, abdominal pain, straining at stool, and fever. Although it tends to occur more in the summer months, it may occur anywhere and at any time of the year. The digestive tract remains very sensitive for a long time, and diet must be carefully regulated for months after recovery from the acute infection.

There is *serious danger of dehydration* because of the loss of fluid through diarrhea, and *so your doctor must supervise your child's treatment* and make sure that she is receiving enough fluids, giving them intravenously if necessary.

Diet

In general, a low-residue, low-fat diet is called for (see Table 15, page 179). Infants should be fed sufficiently to meet their nutritional requirements, but they should not be forced to take more food than their limited digestive capacity will permit. There may also be marked loss of appetite with dysentery.

Breast-fed infants may continue to nurse at four-hour intervals, with nursing preceded by giving boiled water with a little blackstrap molasses to decrease the intake of milk and avoid the fat-rich last portions of the breast milk. Supplementary fluids should be given every hour, consisting of boiled water, barley or rice water, or very weak herb tea with added blackstrap molasses. In severe cases with vomiting, discontinue nursing for twenty-four hours and give your baby water with blackstrap molasses every hour, *with your doctor giving additional fluids as required.*

Bottle-fed infants should be given skimmed acid milk with added blackstrap molasses. Feedings should be low in fat and nonirritating to the inflamed digestive tract. If your infant refuses food or vomits persistently, withhold all food for twenty-four hours, giving fluids every hour. It is very important to maintain this fluid intake; it may be given in the same forms suggested above for breast-fed infants. *If you can't induce your infant to take enough fluids by mouth, your doctor will have to give them by other means.*

Older infants may be given low-residue foods in addition to the acid-milk mixture, such as gruels of barley flour, cornstarch, arrowroot, farina, or rice. Whole-grain cereals should not be given. Raw ripe apple, scraped to a pulp, or ripe raw or baked banana may be given in increasing amounts, and these are preferable to citrus fruits. Vitamin supplements should also be given, as directed by your pediatrician. If your child refuses acid milk, you may substitute boiled skim milk with or without added blackstrap molasses. Other foods, when eventually added, should be introduced in small amounts.

Older children will also have limited digestive capacity, but aim for a diet that will meet their nutritional needs. You may need to begin by withholding all food for twenty-four hours, giving water with blackstrap molasses hourly to maintain fluid intake. During the first few days give skimmed lactic acid milk, dried or evaporated milk, or boiled skim milk in small amounts every four hours; this may be reinforced with blackstrap molasses. If your child is allergic to cow's milk, use soy, evaporated, or goat's milk. If she won't take milk at all, give gruels of refined cereals such as cornstarch, rice, farina, arrowroot, or barley flour. Fruit might include ripe baked banana or whole or grated raw or baked apple, alternating with herb tea or skimmed broth. As her tolerance to foods returns, make gradual additions such as stewed and strained fruits and vegetables, soft cooked egg, finely chopped meat, toast, arrowroot, or rice crackers, restricting the diet to low-residue, fat-free foods until all symptoms of irritation have cleared.

Herbal Preparations

Any of the following herbs may be used to prepare a tea that will help with the diarrhea of dysentery:

Red Raspberry (leaf) or *Wintergreen*	Place ½ teaspoon of selected herb in a pot. Add 1 cup freshly boiled water. Cover and steep for 5–10 minutes. Drink warm.
or *Barberry* or *Licorice* or *Madder* or *Pomegranate* or *Red Raspberry* (root bark) or *Sumac* berries	Add ½ teaspoon of selected herb to 1½ pints boiling water. Cover and continue boiling at a slow boil for about 30 minutes. Allow to cool slowly in the closed container. Drink cold, one swallow or one tablespoon at a time.

EARACHE
See Herbal Remedies under OTITIS MEDIA

ECZEMA

This troublesome allergic skin eruption may appear soon after birth in infants who are receiving breast or cow's milk. Beginning as a mild red rash, usually on the face, it may go on to form deeper red, itchy patches, which begin to ooze if your baby scratches them, eventually forming crusts. The cause is generally an allergenic food in the baby's diet, although contact with irritating substances, such as wool, and climatic conditions may also play an inciting or aggravating role. *Your doctor will need to investigate the source of the problem* and will recommend local treatment for the skin, as well as ways of avoiding irritating substances. This can be a maddening condition for both baby and parents. Generally, infantile eczemas eventually clear up; in the meantime, a patient and consistent control of your infant's diet is required.

Diet

As with asthma and other allergic problems, your breast-fed infant may be receiving an allergenic substance in the breast milk. If skin-testing on your baby reveals specific foods to which he is sensitive, these should be eliminated from the mother's diet, as should commonly allergenic foods such as wheat, egg, and chocolate, and rather than drink whole cow's milk the mother should eat a cup of yogurt at each meal. The nursing mother must avoid any food that has been known in the past to produce digestive or allergic problems in her baby, and should avoid constipation, which may occur on her restricted diet. (See "Constipation" for some herbal laxatives; double the specified dosage to determine adult dose.) It is important to avoid overfeeding your baby and to provide only the amount of calories actually required; the amount taken may be decreased by giving him a little water before each nursing, offering only one breast each time, and limiting feedings to eight minutes at four-hour intervals. Additional nutrients must be added to the allergic breast-fed infant's diet with great caution, and vitamin supplements will be needed to ensure proper nutrition, but be sure to avoid any with artificial coloring or flavoring. Vitamin C may be provided in the form of orange juice that has been strained through fine mesh to remove all traces of rind, which contains potentially irritating volatile oils; if this still makes the eczema worse, then try lemon, grapefruit, or tomato juice in gradually increasing amounts. Or the vitamin-C tonic described on page 147 may be helpful, if your child isn't allergic to any of the ingredients. Other foods may similarly be added cautiously to the breast-fed baby's diet, in the same manner as for bottle-fed infants.

For bottle-fed babies the most common cause of eczema is sensitivity to cow's milk. Your doctor may recommend switching to other forms of milk such as goat's or soy milk or evaporated milk. Allergy to sugars is not as common, but it is another possibility to be explored. In changing sugars in your baby's formula, remember that honey may not be a good substitute since many infants are allergic to the pollens in honey; and if honey is tolerated, be sure it is given only *boiled* to infants. A formula of evaporated cow's or goat's milk or soy milk, with 10 percent added nonallergenic sugar, such as blackstrap molasses, given every four hours, might be the final diet. Have your doctor help determine the appropriate amount, since overfeeding must be avoided. The low sugar content of such a formula produces a mild dehydration that will help with the oozing form of eczema, especially if salt and fluids are also limited. Other foods such as fruits, vegetables, and cereals must be added very cautiously to make up your infant's nutrient requirements, using supplements as necessary to ensure proper nutrition; *consult your doctor* as to which supplements are needed, and in what quantities.

For older children with allergic eczema, an adequate diet can be constructed by reviewing your child's feeding history, the results of skin tests, and trials of various foods. Your child's likes and dislikes must be considered, since children are often found to be allergic to the very foods they have an instinctive distaste for. A trial of various foods is done by placing your child on an elimination diet for a week (see "Allergy"), giving only those foods to which he has shown negative skin tests and no previous suspected allergic reaction. If the eczema improves, continue to add other test-negative foods; if there is no improvement, put your child on soy milk for a week, adding a single nonallergenic food at a time and determining its effect before adding anything else. *Your doctor will need to supervise this process,* and, needless to say, much loving encouragement will be in order to help your child through this trying period of food restriction. Eventually you should be able to build up a balanced, nonallergenic diet, ensuring proper caloric intake by adding sweetener, starch, or oil.

Herbal Preparations

An *external* application to relieve the inflammation of eczema may be prepared of *goldenseal.* Add ¼ teaspoon of the powdered root to 1 pint of boiling water; cover and boil slowly for 30 minutes. Let cool slowly in the covered container and apply topically to affected area.

EPILEPSY

In recent years a number of potent drugs have been introduced in the treatment of the various forms of this convulsive disorder. Interestingly, before such drugs were developed the treatment of choice was through diet, namely the use of ketogenic (ketone-producing) diets. Of course, the diagnosis and treatment of childhood epilepsy must always be *supervised by your pediatrician;* but it is noteworthy that current medical thinking appears to be coming full circle and returning to a dietary approach once again. While *we cannot here recommend a diet for home treatment of childhood epilepsy,* the following information may open up a fruitful line for your physician to explore further.

Diet

Current therapy in treating seizures in childhood epilepsy consists of ketogenic diets. The strategy here is to use fats as the principal source of energy, and reduce the ingestion of carbohydrates to a bare minimum. It has been known since at least 1921 that ketogenic diets would reduce seizures in epilepsy; however, the way diets were constructed in the past was of course based on foods themselves, usually consisting of long-chain fats. In our technological age, today's food scientists have devised compounds called MCTs, or medium-chain triglycerides, which consist of fats with medium chain lengths, as opposed to fats of long chain lengths. It is claimed that by using MCTs as the principal food source, the child is less likely to develop an adverse reaction. However, it should be remembered that MCT oil very frequently causes diarrhea, which is certainly an undesirable side effect; besides, it is very expensive. In addition, such a ketogenic diet based upon a synthetic oil is not adequate in vitamins and minerals. Nevertheless, the strategy of using a ketogenic diet should be reinforced as a rational method of treating epilepsy in children.

A "modern" diet for treating epilepsy using MCT consists of supplying 50 percent to 70 percent of the total calories using MCT oil, limiting protein content to 10 percent of the total caloric intake, and limiting carbohydrates to 19 percent of the total caloric intake. Fats other than MCTs are limited to 11 percent of the total caloric intake. Thus, a typical 1500-calorie diet for an adolescent child consists of a disproportionate amount of MCT oil (9 tablespoons), two vegetable exchanges, one fruit exchange, one bread exchange, three medium fat exchanges from meats, and one additional fat exchange. In addition, vitamin and mineral supplements are required.

Prior to the development of MCT oil and the total synthetic approach to the treatment of childhood epilepsy, Dr. Kugelmass recommended a carefully calculated set of ketogenic diets, adjusting the ratio of ketogenic (ketone-producing) and antiketogenic (ketone-inhibiting) foods according to the degree of ketosis desired for control of the epilepsy. Essentially, fats are ketogenic, yielding largely ketogenic substances; carbohydrates are antiketogenic, and proteins fall in between:

$$
\begin{array}{rl}
1 \text{ gm. fat yields} & 0.9 \text{ gm. ketogenic } + \\
& 0.1 \text{ gm. antiketogenic substances} \\
1 \text{ gm. carbohydrate yields} & 1 \text{ gm. antiketogenic substances} \\
1 \text{ gm. protein yields} & 0.46 \text{ gm. ketogenic } + \\
& 0.58 \text{ gm. antiketogenic substances}
\end{array}
$$

Thus, for a given total caloric intake, the component nutrients can be adjusted to make the diet more or less ketogenic.

A sample 1500-calorie diet from Dr. Kugelmass's regimen, designed for a six-year-old and having a ketogenic/antiketogenic ratio of 3:1, is given in Table 21, for the purpose of illustration only. Obviously, *if you desire to explore this time-tested dietary approach for control of epilepsy, you will need to do so under the very close supervision of your pediatrician.*

Herbal Preparations

Gentle herbal teas, long valued for their antispasmodic (anticonvulsant) properties, may be made from any one of the following:

Passionflower or *Chamomile* or *Scullcap*	Place ½ teaspoon of selected herb in a pot. Add 1 cup freshly boiled water. Cover and steep for 5–10 minutes. Drink warm.

A stronger relaxing tea may be made using *valerian,* ½ teaspoon of the root to 1 cup of water, steeped for 5–10 minutes. Use *fresh* plant material only!

FEVER

Of course, fever can have many causes, and your doctor will need to determine the underlying disorder. In all fevers associated with infectious diseases, however, you will encounter similar feeding problems, which will need to be dealt with in order to maintain your child's nutritional status. Especially during the early stages of any feverish complaint, your child may have a loss of appetite, nausea, vomiting, and/or diarrhea. Anemia may develop, as may disturbances in the electrolyte and water balance. During fever, salt is retained in the body tissues, with accompanying water retention. At the end of a febrile period, your child's body loses salt and water, resulting in a sudden loss of weight. Once you understand the reason for this, it should not be a cause for undue

TABLE 21
Ketogenic Diet*
6-year-old child
1500 calories
(NOTE: Sample diet only; *not* for use in feeding!)

Prot.: 41.0 gm. Ketogenic/Antiketogenic = 3:1
Fat: 143.2 gm.
Carb.: 11.1 gm.

Foods	Amount	Gm.	Prot.	Fat	Carb.
Breakfast					
Strawberries	3 T†	45	0.4	0.3	2.7
Cream, 40%	2 T	30	0.6	12.2	0.4
Egg	1	50	6.0	5.0	—
Bacon, crisp	2 str.	20	4.0	10.0	—
Bran wafers					
Butter	½ pat	5	—	4.2	—
Cod-liver oil	2 t	10	—	10.0	—
Dinner					
Lamb chop, broiled	1 lg.	60	13.2	18.0	—
Turnip, mashed	2 T	30	0.4	—	2.0
Butter	1 pat	10	—	8.4	—
Cranberries, strained	5 t	25	—	—	2.0
Bran biscuit					
Butter	2 pats	20	—	16.8	—
Cream, 40%	2 T	30	2.4	12.2	0.4
Water	2 T	30			
Casec (casein)	2 gm.	2			
Supper					
Beef liver, chopped	3 T	45	9.9	4.5	1.4
Egg yolk	1	15	3.0	5.0	—
Bone marrow	1 T	15	0.3	14.0	—
Watercress	10 pcs.	25	0.4	—	0.7
Mayonnaise	1 T	15	—	11.7	—
Bran biscuit					
Butter	2½ T	13	—	10.9	—
Rhubarb, strained	4 T	60	0.4	—	1.5

*After Kugelmass (1940).
†Capital *T* is for *tablespoon;* lower case t, teaspoon.

alarm. Remember that fevers will go up at night. *Be sure to check with your doctor,* however, to determine what temperature is the danger signal at which you must call immediately for emergency treatment. The vitamin-C "cocktail" described on page 147 will be helpful in fevers due to viral infections.

Diet

With fever, the total metabolic rate of your child's body increases by 7 percent for every degree Fahrenheit increase in body temperature. Moreover, the increased metabolic demands during fever lead to a destruction of protein in the body. The best protection against excessive destruction of body tissue during infectious diseases with fever is to feed your child a high-calorie, high-protein diet. Thus the old folk adage "Feed a fever" has a basis in fact. Unfortunately, although your child's food requirements are increased during the course of fever, her appetite and digestive capacity may be reduced. Feeding strategies are therefore based on getting adequate supplies of nutrients into your child without aggravating digestive troubles.

You may continue to nurse your breast-fed baby, decreasing the nursing time as dictated by her appetite, nursing at only one breast for several minutes at a time. To ensure adequate fluid intake, give water in increased amounts between feedings. For bottle-fed infants also you will likely need to reduce the feedings at the beginning of the feverish episode, by keeping up the regular formula schedule but eliminating other added foods. If there is digestive upset, you may switch to another type of milk, or change the formula entirely if digestive problems are severe. Maintain fluid intake by giving increased quantities of water and fruit juices at frequent intervals. As the fever subsides, digestive problems should clear, and you may reintroduce the original nursing schedule or diet for your breast- or bottle-fed baby. Remember that with acute illnesses, it's not so important to maintain the usual total food intake as it is to provide lots of fluids and feedings rich in readily digestible carbohydrate. Forcing unwanted food on your baby will only increase the chances of digestive problems. During fever in *chronic* infectious illnesses, on the other hand, your infant must be encouraged to maintain a proper intake of nutrients even if she has no appetite. Use concentrated-milk mixtures, adding semisolid food and fruit juices between feedings.

Older children's nutritional needs during fever are primarily for water, electrolytes, and readily available sources of energy, so they should be given lots of liquids, including water, and easily digestible sugars. The proportion of nutrients should be about 10 percent protein, 70 percent carbohydrate, and the rest consisting of alkali-forming fruits and vegetables (see Table 16, page 184). A diet rich in readily digestible carbohydrates is the best protection against excessive protein loss in your child's body. Most fevers will break in 24–48 hours, and it isn't

TABLE 22
Liquid Diet*

Soups	Milks
Milk soups, strained	Skimmed milk
Meat juice	Whole milk
Meat broths, strained	Yogurt or other fermented dairy products
	Goat's milk
Cereals	Soy milk
Thin cereal gruels, strained	Malted milk (no artificial
	color or flavor)
Beverages	
Fruit juices	
Herb teas	

*After Kugelmass (1940).

TABLE 23
Soft Diet*

Soups	Fruits and Vegetables
Milk soups	Stewed mild fruits, no skins
Meat juice	or seeds
Meat broths	Vegetables, pureed
Cereals and Breads	**Desserts**
Toast, thin, crisp	Gelatin (flavored with fruit
Toast, in milk	juice; no artificial color
Cereals, well cooked	or flavor)
	Junket (flavored with fruit
Dairy Products	juice; no artificial color
Eggs, soft-cooked	or flavor)
Cottage cheese	Custard
Yogurt	Cereal puddings
Butter	Ice cream

*After Kugelmass (1940).

practical to try to force-feed a child who is feeling completely awful. Keep up the liquids and the vitamin-C tonic if viral infection is suspected, while keeping your child
covered loosely with cotton pajamas and a light blanket
to prevent either accidental chill or overheating.

A child with a *chronic* febrile infection will require a
high-calorie diet. You must make every effort to persuade her to take the foods she needs. You may give a liquid diet (Table 22) to begin with, and gradually increase
the caloric content by progressing to a soft diet (Table
23) and then a complete diet, with slightly higher than
normal protein content and maximum carbohydrate content, by the end of the illness. By that time fat should be
well tolerated, and may be given in large amounts. Of

course, throughout the course of the illness you will need to provide fluids in large quantities. Even if your child is vomiting, you may offer food again a few minutes after vomiting and it can probably be kept down. (See Tables 22 and 23 for foods included in liquid and soft diets; you may be able to make some additions from the recipes in Book IV.)

Herbal Preparations

Choose any *one* of the following herbs for a good tea for relieving fever:

Balm	Place ½ teaspoon of selected herb
or *Boneset*	in a pot. Add 1 cup freshly boiled
or *Buckbean*	water. Cover and steep for 5–10
or *Feverfew*	minutes. Drink warm.
or *Yarrow*	

Magnolia Bark	Add ½ teaspoon of selected herb to
or *Sarsaparilla*	1½ pints boiling water. Cover and
or *Willow Bark*	continue boiling at a slow boil for
(*White or Black*)	about 30 minutes. Allow to cool
	slowly in the closed container.
	Drink cold, one swallow or 1
	tablespoon at a time.

FLATULENCE

Gas may accumulate in your child's intestinal tract owing to air-swallowing, or because of fermentation of carbohydrates or putrefaction of proteins in the intestines. With the accumulation of gas in the bowel, there will be the occasional expulsion of flatus. Prolonged distension of the bowel can lead to more serious problems, and so *with your doctor's assistance* it is important to determine the source of the problem.

Diet

The condition can usually be cleared by giving a diet low in fat and high in fluids, free from allergy-producing or irritating foods. Table 24 lists common foods that are likely to produce flatulence, and those that help prevent it.

TABLE 24
Relation of Foods to Flatulence*

Flatulence-Producing Foods	Flatulence-Preventing Foods
Fruits and Vegetables	**Fruits and Vegetables**
Raw fruits	Fruit juice
Raisins	Stewed fruit
Nuts	Peas
Cabbage	Carrots
Broccoli	Beets
Beans	Potatoes
Turnips	
Protein Foods	**Protein Foods**
Cheeses	Milk
Meat broths	Cottage cheese
Stews	Eggs
	Meat
	Fish
Sugars	Chicken
Sweet foods	
	Cereals and Breads
	Dry Toast
	Cream of wheat
	Oatmeal

*After Kugelmass (1940).

Herbal Preparations

The following herbs are gently soothing for children of all ages, including infants:

Chamomile
or *Anise*
or *Fennel*

Place ½ teaspoon of selected herb in a pot. Add 1 cup freshly boiled water. Steep for 5–10 minutes. Drink warm. (May be flavored with 1 *hibiscus* leaf.)

See also COLIC

FLU
See COLDS *for general procedures in mild viral illnesses*

FOOD POISONING

Food poisoning can occur as a result of bacterial contamination of foods, chemical poisons, or poisonous substances produced by bacteria. The most common cause is infection of foods with salmonella bacteria, which may grow in foods that have not been properly refrigerated or that have been prepared hours before serving, and so picnics and party dishes are among the common sources of food poisoning. Proper cooking is the best safeguard against salmonella contamination.

The first symptoms of bacterial food infection usually come on suddenly six to twenty-four hours after the contaminated food is eaten. Severe, crampy abdominal pain may be the first symptom, followed by nausea, vomiting, and diarrhea. With food poisoning from chemicals or bacterial toxins (such as botulism), there is usually constipation. *In any case of suspected food poisoning, your doctor should be called immediately;* this is particularly important in the case of suspected chemical or bacterial toxin poisoning, which must be treated medically on an emergency basis.

Diet

If your child is having abdominal distress that you suspect is due to the eating of some food, withhold all food for twenty-four hours, giving only fluids by mouth as tolerated. If vomiting is present, your doctor may decide to give additional fluids by artificial means. Once the acute attack has subsided you may begin to add foods gradually, but be careful not to force your child to eat more than she can tolerate. There has been injury to her digestive tract, and it will not return to full, efficient function for days or weeks. Attempting to return to a full diet too quickly will only prolong digestive upset and delay recovery. At first, feed your child only strained fruit juices, raw apples or ripe bananas, well-cooked cereals, soft white rice, mashed boiled white or sweet potato, or crackers mashed in chicken broth. Avoid whole milk, but fermented milk may be given, preferably low-fat or skimmed, such as low-fat acidophilus milk. Tender meats such as fish and chicken (all fat removed) may next be added to the diet. All foods should be bland and smooth. Such a low-residue diet will not produce much stool; don't be tempted to give a laxative to stimulate bowel function.

Herbal Preparations

To induce vomiting of recently eaten food that is suspected of being contaminated, give *ipecac* syrup, according to label directions.

Safe and soothing herbal remedies for stomach upset, which may be given to infants as well as older children, include:

Chamomile or *Fennel*	Place ½ teaspoon of selected herb in a pot. Add 1 cup freshly boiled water. Cover and steep for 5–10 minutes. Drink warm.

A stronger remedy, recommended only for children over ten years old, is *gotu kola*, ¼ teaspoon to 1 cup of water, prepared in the same manner as described above.

GAS
See COLIC; FLATULENCE

GASTRITIS, ACUTE

This inflammation of the mucous lining of the stomach is often confused with indigestion, but indigestion doesn't produce inflammation of the mucosa. Symptoms of gastritis may include loss of appetite, a sensation of pressure and fullness in the upper mid-abdomen, nausea, headache, and vomiting, sometimes of bloody material. Possible causes include infection, food poisoning, spicy or allergenic foods, chemicals, or drugs. Of course, you must eliminate the possibility of accidental poisoning owing to a harmful chemical, drug, or bacterial toxin. If such poisoning is suspected, *call your physician immediately* to pursue emergency treatment. Once you have ruled out poisoning, other cases of gastritis will generally clear up after 24–48 hours if the offending substance is eliminated from your child's intake.

Diet

During the first twenty-four hours, your child should receive no food, with fluid needs being supplied in the form of cracked ice or sips of water by mouth. *Your doctor may need to give additional fluids by artificial means.*

When feeding is begun, start with bland fluids such as skim milk with lime water, vegetable broths thickened with cereal, rice, or gelatin, going on when tolerated to a soft diet of thin cereal gruels, vegetable purees, soft white rice, mashed boiled sweet or white potato, crackers mashed in chicken broth, stewed fruits, custards, ice cream, yogurt, and milk drinks.

Herbal Preparations

Any of the following herbs may be used to prepare a soothing tea for irritated stomach:

Angelica	Place ½ teaspoon of selected herb
or *Chamomile*	in a pot. Add 1 cup freshly boiled
or *Dandelion*	water. Cover and steep for 5–10
or *Holy Thistle*	minutes. Drink warm.
or *Peppermint*	

HAY FEVER

Hay fever is characterized by recurrent or persistent attacks of sneezing with stuffy, itching nose, with watery discharge. Hay fever differs from the common cold in that attacks are short in duration and are not accompanied by more generalized symptoms of illness. The disorder may be seasonal, and is brought on by an allergenic substance, the most common offenders being inhaled substances such as house dust or seasonal pollens. Next in importance are foods, the most frequent provokers of hay fever being wheat, egg, milk, fish, nuts, chocolate, buckwheat, celery, beans, potato, and banana. Other possible contributing factors are drugs, bacteria, and changes in weather. *Your doctor will need to determine the causative factor,* perhaps by performing skin tests. If these reveal nothing helpful, it may be necessary to look for food allergens by doing diet tests such as those described under "Allergy," based on your child's dietary history and his likes and dislikes in foods. Your doctor will supervise the use of medications for an acute attack of hay fever; remember that it's wise to avoid using excessive quantities of antihistamines or sprays since these powerful medicines may set up a tissue reaction worse than the original problem.

Diet

Diet in hay fever should avoid all foods that commonly incite attacks, such as those listed above, unless testing has shown them to be safe. All foods should be cooked, and any vitamin deficiencies from the restricted diet should be made up with supplements; *ask your pediatrician what your child should be taking in addition to her usual supplement formula.* The diet should be acid-forming—that is, high in protein, low in fruits and vegetables (see Table 16, page 184)—minimal in salt, sugar, and water, in order to reduce the level of fluid in body tissues, since excessive fluid in tissues increases allergic reactivity. Once it has been determined what foods if any are causing the hay fever, your child should be put on a balanced diet excluding these allergenic foods for long enough to produce desensitization. In general, food-incited hay fever is easier to treat than hay fever due to inhalants or other causes. If it's not possible to eliminate completely the offending food, it will be necessary to do other sorts of desensitization treatments. Your doctor will supervise these treatments and the control of your child's environment to eliminate exposure to allergenic substances.

Herbal Preparations

Herbal Vaporizer Mix. Use vaporizer at night to relieve congestion. The herbal mix consists of ½ ounce each of *boneset, burdock,* and *eucalyptus.* Place herbs in a cheesecloth bag and boil for 20 minutes in 2 quarts of water. Strain. Place in vaporizer, then dilute with water to reach proper level. Let steam all night near child.

Used singly, either of the following herbs will help relieve hay-fever symptoms:

Ephedra
or *Grindelia*

Place ½ teaspoon of selected herb in a pot. Add 1 cup freshly boiled water. Cover and steep for 5–10 minutes. Drink warm.

For children who are not allergic to it, we also recommend that they eat *bee pollen,* the richest natural source of vitamin B_6.

See also ALLERGY

HEADACHE
See MIGRAINE *for herbal remedies;*
also HYPOGLYCEMIA
(one possible cause of headache)

HYPERACTIVITY (Hyperkinesis)

If Tom Sawyer were alive today and in grade school, no doubt he would be declared a "hyperactive child" by a teacher eager to subdue him. To apply a medical term to social behavior is the road to *1984* and all the implied dangers of mind control and psychoactive drugs. I have long felt that teachers who recommend Ritalin and other forms of "speed"-like drugs to control our children (whose attention they should be able to engage through exciting teaching!) ought to be threatened with legal action from parents on the premise that teachers are not licensed to practice medicine and make diagnoses!

Diet

Dr. Ben Feingold accepts that there is such a disorder as hyperkinesis (the British do not), and he recommends a diet that contains no salicylates, artificial colors, or artificial flavors, because he believes that these compounds are the agents that incite the disorder. More recently, Dr. Feingold has extended his list of food additives suspected as causative agents to include BHA and BHT, two antioxidants commonly used by food manufacturers to extend shelf life. While the Feingold diet is reputed to help between 40 and 70 percent of children who follow its prescriptions, experiments are equivocal. Nevertheless, as I learned in elementary biology, "When the animal and the drawing disagree, the animal is always right." Thus, if this reasonable diet that does away with offensive food additives brings relief to a sizable number of children, if only because of "family dynamics, increased attention, placebo effect, or a change in nutritional status" (*Nutrition and the M.D.*, Vol. VI, January, 1980), we must agree with Dr. Feingold's drug-free approach.

Foods to eliminate from your child's diet include those that contain natural salicylates. These include tomatoes, cucumbers, apples, apricots, cherries, grapes, grape drinks, raisins, wine, nectarines, oranges, peaches, plums, and prunes. Almonds and some other nuts are also forbidden. In addition, all foods containing artificial colors and flavors, as well as the antioxidants BHT and BHA, are also to be avoided.

You will also want to watch out for medicines and vitamins made with artificial colors and flavors, toothpastes, tooth powders, antacids, perfumes, cough drops, mouthwash, and aspirin. As for herbal teas, remember that willow bark was used for centuries to reduce fevers owing to its aspirinlike effects. This is due to naturally occurring salicylates, and so this herb must *not* be used if you suspect that your child is "hyperactive."

From my own experience as a parent and clinical nutritionist, I suspect that much of the "crazy" behavior of children (my own included) follows too much sucrose, television, and plain old boredom. Go out for a walk or a run with your child each day for a month and see what that does for both your dispositions!

Herbal Preparations

As explained above, *willow bark* is to be *avoided*, because of the salicylates it contains.

For insomnia and restlessness, a mixture of *passionflower* and *chamomile* has long been used in Italy. The herbs may be prepared singly as follows:

Passionflower may be used in the *tincture* form. For children, the dose is 1–2 drops of the tincture in a glass of water. If the *herb* is used, place ¼ to ½ teaspoon in a pot and add 1 cup freshly boiled water. Cover and steep for 5–10 minutes. Drink warm.

Chamomile tea may be prepared using ½ teaspoon of the flowers, steeped in a cup of freshly boiled water for 5–10 minutes. Drink warm.

HYPOGLYCEMIA

"I believe in the immortality of the soul periodically. My opinions depend entirely on my physical condition. According to whether I have greater or lesser vitality, or my digestion is functioning well or badly, or the atmosphere I breathe is thick or thin, or the food I eat is light or heavy, I am a Spinozist, a Socinian, or a Catholic, unbelieving or devout."

MONTESQUIEU, Persian Letter

No illness is more subject to skepticism in the medical profession than hypoglycemia. This disorder is commonly alluded to as the "nonillness" of the decade. For many, many years, while nutritionists have vociferously argued that reactive hypoglycemia, or low blood sugar, explains the symptoms expressed by so many patients, doctors have mistakenly diagnosed this all-too-common disorder as mental retardation, or neurosis, or schizophrenia, diabetes, alcoholism, menopause, Parkinson's syndrome, rheumatoid arthritis, bronchial asthma, cerebral arteriosclerosis, hyperinsulinism, neurodermatitis, Ménière's syndrome, and others.

One of the great pioneers in this field is Carlton Fredericks, Ph.D., whose book *Low Blood Sugar and You* is an absolute must for anyone who suspects he or she may be suffering from this disorder. This fact-filled book reports on the original work done in this area by Dr. Seale Harris, which appeared in the *Journal of the American Medical Association* in 1924, and later work by Dr. Stephen Gyland, who himself was plagued by symptoms he was unable to diagnose; namely, "unprovoked anxieties, tremors, weakness, dizziness, faintness, paroxysmal tachycardia, and difficulties with concentration and memory." According to Dr. Fredericks, Dr. Gyland went from one physician to another, and was diagnosed as having a brain tumor by one, diabetes by another, cerebral arteriosclerosis by another, and so on. Dr. Gyland, still unable to work and not having found the physician who could treat him, somehow fortuituously found Dr. Harris's original paper and ordered for himself the six-hour glucose-tolerance test. By analyzing the results, he decided that he did have low blood sugar, or reactive hypoglycemia, and when he followed the correct diet, his symptoms all but disappeared. Dr. Gyland not only cured himself, but treated many, many hundreds of patients for hypoglycemia, eventually publishing a definitive paper on the subject.

Do any of these symptoms fit you or your child? If so, you *may* be suffering from low blood sugar:

nervousness, irritability, exhaustion, faintness, dizziness, tremor, cold sweats, weak spells, depression, vertigo, drowsiness, headaches, digestive disturbances, forgetfulness, insomnia, constant worrying, mental confusion, internal trembling, heart palpitation, muscular pain, numbness, asocial, antisocial, or unsocial behavior, indecisiveness, crying spells, loss of sex drive in females, allergies, incoordination, leg cramps, poor concentration, blurred vision, twitching and jerking of muscles, itching and crawling sensations on the skin, gasping for breath, smothering spells, staggering, sighing and yawning, male impotence, unconsciousness, night terrors, nightmares, rheumatoid arthritis, phobias, neurodermatitis, suicidal intent, nervous breakdown, convulsions.

These symptoms are clearly of the nature that "neurotics" seem to suffer from, and are therefore largely laughed at or treated with chagrin by too many practitioners; but I can assure you from my own experience that these symptoms are no laughing matter to a person who has seen anywhere from two to six physicians, many of whom are specialists, who have subjected him to some of the most costly and unnecessary tests, while all the time treating them as though they were a joke. Yet, all serious symptoms *should* be referred to a physician.

Not long ago I had a patient who had been on disability insurance for over eight years, yet back in 1970 this man had been earning over $40,000 a year as a corporate executive. When he first came to my office, he had a hangdog look, was very suspicious, uncommunicative, didn't really want to trust what we were talking about, and was altogether unenthusiastic. He told me that he had been on disability for all of these years, and had already been to see six physicians who had misdiagnosed his illness. The reason he knew that his illness had been misdiagnosed was because the suggested treatments never eliminated his chronic fatigue, his inability to concentrate, his indecisiveness, etc. In fact, this poor man told me that occasionally he would go into a supermarket and begin crying in the aisles because he was unable to decide between one breakfast cereal and another! He would then often run back to his room and sit there for the rest of the day. Typically, also, this patient drank anywhere from ten to twelve cups of coffee daily, and craved carbohydrates, particularly pastries.

Well, as we normally do in cases such as this, a six-hour glucose-tolerance test was ordered, and the results were analyzed. Now, many physicians who are beginning to become aware that reactive hypoglycemia may be a true epidemic in a sucrose- and refined-carbohydrate-ridden society will order this test. Unfortunately, they do not interpret the results correctly. Dr. Gyland tells us that a final blood-glucose reading that drops below the initial fasting level by as little as 10 mg% is a meaningful diagnosis of low blood sugar. Most physicians set a standard for low blood sugar as any level below 50 mg%. Of course, the best answer is this: follow the appropriate diet. If the symptoms disappear, then you can be sure that the diagnosis of low blood sugar is confirmed.

There is of course a quick test that requires much less time that can also be used with an amazing degree of accuracy. This is reported by Dr. Fredericks:

> Basically, the Goodman test calls for a determination of the fasting blood sugar level before breakfast. The patient is then instructed to eat his normal breakfast, and the test is repeated 45 minutes to one hour later. If the blood sugar at that time has not risen 50 percent or more above the fasting level, the patient is hypoglycemic, and this is true even though the initial and the second readings both fall within "normal range." This may be compared with the long test, in which many blood sugar levels are determined over a six-hour period after sugar has been fed as a challenge to the pancreas.

The above values and test criteria are for adults. Exact values for determining whether your child may be hypoglycemic have not been established, and for this reason it may be safer if you suspect this disorder to follow the recommended diet, because this diet is not only useful in controlling hypoglycemia but is also a reasonable way of feeding children. Basically, it consists of the following.

Diet

Eat protein-rich foods such as poultry that has been skinned, fish, or lean meat. If not allergic to milk and dairy, cottage cheese and other cheese are also valuable food sources. (Fried food is to be avoided; the frying creates a thick skin, which decreases digestibility.) When it comes to vegetables, the following are allowed: broccoli, chard, cabbage, cucumbers, cauliflower, eggplant, spinach, lettuce, tomato, string beans, and kale. Allowable fruits include apples, berries, melons, pears, and peaches; these must be fresh or frozen, but by no means are fruits in heavy syrup allowed. Also, avoid all dried fruit that has been candied. Oranges and grapefruit are allowed, but only in moderation. Allowable carbohydrates include all unrefined carbohydrates.* I repeat: you will probably find recommendations that hypoglycemics avoid all carbohydrates, or severely limit them! This is unfortunately very misleading. Unrefined carbohydrates, such as true whole grains, potatoes, sweet potatoes, lentils, legumes, and so on, of the type found in Book IV, are highly recommended. You see, while refined carbohydrates such as white flour or pasta made from white flour, or, worse still, sucrose, glucose, or fructose, are like drugs to most people, but particularly to hypoglycemics, on the other hand unrefined carbohydrates are slow-burning fuels that metabolize more slowly and give the person a better "glow" for a longer period of time.

Foods absolutely to be forbidden include any made with sugar, such as cakes, pies, cookies, chewing gum, candy, pizza, matzoh, crackers, sauces, gravies, ketchup, and dressings containing flour. All of these foods, *repeat,* must be avoided like the plague! Liquids absolutely for-

---

*Diabetics have an additional problem and should see the entry on diabetes.

bidden include all soft drinks, including diet soft drinks, any other fruit drinks that may be made with corn-syrup sweetener, fructose, glucose, or sucrose, and of course beverages that contain caffeine, such as colas, cocoas, chocolates, black tea, and coffee. Alcoholic beverages, needless to say, are also forbidden.

Of critical importance is *when* these foods are eaten. The hypoglycemic must eat six small meals per day, rather than the usual three large meals. This better enables the utilization of foods and tends to stabilize blood sugar.

To summarize: diets that are rich in complex carbohydrates and fiber are the goal, and low-carbohydrate diets, which are usually prescribed for hypoglycemia, should be totally eliminated. By feeding your child from the recipes provided in Book IV, and augmenting these diets with lean meat, skinned poultry, fish, and dairy (provided you do not adhere to the vegetarian regimen, or your child is not allergic to milk products), you will achieve the benefits you are seeking. As one who suffered from severe, debilitating migraine headaches for seventeen years, and who was misdiagnosed by too many physicians over too many years, I can personally tell you that by experimenting with my own diet after leaving home, and having discovered that sugar was the culprit, and having made the proper dietary adjustments, my migraine headaches, which had been the biggest problem in my life, miraculously disappeared.

As a final note, let me tell you this. Many people begin with all good intentions and follow the hypoglycemic diet rigorously and achieve great results, usually an abatement of all symptoms. Unfortunately, after one or two months they are feeling so good and so high that they begin to "cheat," and the results are quite dramatic. As I tell these people in advance: arsenic is arsenic; a little arsenic is of no benefit to your body. It's the same with refined carbohydrates, caffeine, and alcohol, and skipping meals for the hypoglycemic; a little bit of each of these things is as deadly as a lot, especially during the critical first six months of the dietary regimen. It is true that after the first six months some of these items can be added back in small quantities, but this must be done very cautiously and with the guidance of a competent nutritionist.

Herbal Preparations

For the anxiety and insomnia that often accompany hypoglycemia, a gently soothing tea may be made of either of the following:

Passionflower or *Chamomile*	Place ½ teaspoon of selected herb in a pot. Add 1 cup freshly boiled water. Cover and steep for 5–10 minutes. Drink warm.

For a stronger remedy for the same complaints, use *valerian* root, ½ teaspoon to 1 cup of water, steeped for 5–10 minutes. Use *fresh* plant material only!

INDIGESTION

Indigestion may produce a wide variety of symptoms. Acute attacks usually begin suddenly with loss of appetite, nausea, vomiting, constipation or diarrhea, coated tongue, and foul-smelling breath. With persistent, chronic indigestion, the child, unable to digest and absorb the amounts of food required, becomes malnourished and fails to gain weight properly.

The problem may be in the stomach, perhaps beginning with recurrent bouts of acute gastritis (see "Gastritis"), or it may be in the intestines. The causes may be widely varied also. Among the most common are sensitivity to one or more of the nutrients; the eating of highly seasoned, irritating foods; food allergies; infection; unbalanced diet; and hot weather.

Allergy-prone children tend to have an intolerance

to the protein in cow's milk, which forms tough curds that irritate the digestive tract. Carbohydrate intolerance may lead to a fermentative type of diarrhea, with frothy, acid stools that irritate the mucous membranes. Some children may be intolerant of fat during the early months of life. Treatment of indigestion depends on your doctor's determination of the location and cause of the problem.

Diet

Gastric Indigestion. When the problem is in the stomach (gastric indigestion), infants should be switched to small amounts of easily digested concentrated-milk mixture for prompt relief of symptoms. Generally a formula of 2 percent skim or lactic-acid milk or kefir, with added blackstrap molasses, will be helpful. If cow's milk is not well tolerated, then goat's or soy milk may be begun. Any food that is easily digested may be given, in small amounts only. Sometimes it will help to eliminate a class of nutrients—fat, protein, or sugar—if intolerance is suspected. Once tolerance for food is reestablished, feedings are increased by returning to normal meals in a stepwise fashion, resuming one additional normal meal each successive day.

In older children with chronic gastric indigestion, the first step is to provide rest for the stomach as well as for your child's body and emotions as a whole. While a brief period of withholding all food would ordinarily be the best means to clear the stomach, this can't be done in the case of chronic indigestion, because it would aggravate the condition. A bland diet (see Table 25) with limited carbohydrate intake should be begun, giving only skim or fermented milk (such as kefir) at first, then gradually adding thin cereals, strained fruits, and then lean meats, eggs, and strained vegetables. If the stomach contains a lot of mucus, it can be cleared by giving hot drinks (such as herb tea) between meals.

TABLE 25
Bland Foods*

Cereals and Breads	Vegetables	Fats
Cream of Wheat	Potatoes	Cod-liver oil
Arrowroot	Rice	Olive oil
Farina	Spinach	Butter
Oatmeal	Carrots	
Gruel	Green peas	**Desserts**
Crackers	Beets	Puddings:
White bread	Asparagus	Arrowroot
Zwieback		Tapioca
Pasta (noodles, etc.)	**Fluids**	Rice
	Milk:	Cornstarch
Protein Foods	Fresh	Custard
Eggs	Fermented	Junket
Chicken, lean	Evaporated	Ice cream
Fish	Dried	Mousse
	Cream	
	Cream soups	

*After Kugelmass (1940).

Intestinal Indigestion. When the problem is localized to the intestines, the dietary strategy involves the reduction of food intake, with maintenance of fluids. Breast-fed infants with mild indigestion should have their intake of breast milk reduced by cutting the nursing period to 5 minutes at 4-hour intervals; it may be necessary to reduce the total number of breast-feedings as well, alternating with a formula of skimmed lactic-acid milk or boiled skim milk, with or without added blackstrap molasses. When the indigestion is severe and associated with diarrhea, your doctor will likely suspect an infectious disease. Nursing should be discontinued for a period of 12–36 hours, but this doesn't mean your baby should be weaned. During this period, give your infant nothing but water with blackstrap molasses or barley or arrowroot water every hour. After an initial 12–24 hours on this liquid intake, begin to offer small feedings of skimmed lactic-acid milk; if your baby doesn't like the sour taste, try diluted skim milk with blackstrap molasses. On the first day of resuming feedings, to keep formula intake low you may give several ounces of boiled water just before each feeding. During the period when nursing is discontinued, mothers should manually express their breast milk to maintain the flow; a little breast milk may be given boiled or included in the formula. If your infant doesn't respond to this dietary treatment, the intestinal disturbance is probably due to an infectious disorder that *your doctor will need to diagnose and treat.* When normal breast feedings are resumed, if attacks of indigestion occur again, then obviously the mother's diet needs examination, and elimination of offending substances is in order.

Bottle-fed infants with mild cases of intestinal indigestion with diarrhea may be reacting to an unsuitable feeding; your doctor may recommend a dose of castor oil to help clear out the offending food. As with breast-fed babies, several feedings should be omitted and replaced with water with blackstrap molasses or half-strength saline in a blackstrap-molasses solution for twelve hours; then arrowroot, rice or barley water hourly for the next twenty-four hours. After this, previous feedings if suitable may be resumed, but in smaller amounts, at four-hour intervals. It is often helpful to switch temporarily to skimmed lactic-acid milk with blackstrap molasses, or if your baby doesn't like the sour milk, half-strength boiled skim milk with blackstrap molasses, in small amounts. Don't force your baby to take more than she wants, but give extra fluids hourly between feedings. *Severe indigestion with diarrhea will require your doctor's attention,* and if infectious disease is suspected or identified, begin with a twenty-four-hour period of nothing by mouth but hourly fluids, then begin small feedings every four hours. A good formula might be based on skimmed lactic-acid milk, giving about half the usual amount. If your baby takes most of these feedings, you may add carbohydrate in the form of blackstrap molasses. Increase the feedings as your baby's overall health returns, rather than looking for improvement in the stools alone. Once the total volume of food is being taken, you may begin to replace the special feedings with your infant's usual formula, one meal at a time, so that the first day you will give one feeding of the usual formula, two the second day, and so on until all feedings are back to normal, gradually adding other foods as tolerated.

In older children, acute indigestion with diarrhea should be treated as with infants, putting the child to bed and withholding all food for twenty-four hours with only liquids being given at hourly intervals—arrowroot, rice or barley water or warm herb tea, with added blackstrap molasses. Avoid iced drinks, as they stimulate peristalsis. In place of the initial period of food withdrawal, you may give your child several tablespoons of scraped raw apple at hourly intervals for two to three days, along with lots of fluids, and nothing else given by mouth, including medication, for forty-eight hours. When feedings are resumed, you may begin with skimmed broth with rice or barley, refined cereals such as barley, cornstarch, rice, or arrowroot, toast, rice or arrowroot crackers, boiled white potato, ripe banana, or ripe raw apple. Your child will probably not tolerate regular cow's milk well, but acidified milks such as skimmed lactic-acid milk or kefir, with added blackstrap molasses, may be given. Other foods should be added gradually, avoiding those that contain residue until all the symptoms of indigestion and more general infection have cleared up.

Chronic Intestinal Indigestion. *If your baby has recurrent problems with indigestion, your doctor will have to investigate to determine the cause.* In breast-fed babies, one possible cause is *underfeeding.* If this is the problem, you will need to give additional feedings with formula, such as evaporated milk with added blackstrap molasses, with no solid foods given until the indigestion has cleared. Meanwhile, the mother's physical condition and diet should be improved to help increase the milk supply. It may help to eliminate orange juice and cod-liver oil from the baby's diet during the initial period of dietary treatment, adding foods gradually according to tolerance to prevent relapse. If *overfeeding* is producing the indigestion, limit nursing to five minutes or less, offering only one breast at a feeding, at four-hour intervals. If your baby has been getting *excess fat* from the breast milk, shortening the nursing time will eliminate the fat-rich milk at the end of the feeding. Giving your infant several ounces of boiled water just before feeding will also help cut down on breast-milk intake. If your baby continues to be intolerant of breast milk, it may be necessary to express manually, skim partially, and boil the milk, and then feed it at four-hour intervals. The mother's diet may also contain *allergenic substances* that are being passed on to the baby in her milk. Eliminating foods to which the baby shows positive skin tests or other sensitivities, as well as commonly allergenic foods (see Table 11, page 157), may help. If your baby is allergic to a great many foods, then it may be simpler to use formula or soy or evaporated goat's milk. Remember that the breast milk may also contain stimulants or drugs that the mother has been taking, and eliminating these may be enough to clear up your baby's condition. The mother's emotional status can also have an effect on the quality of the milk, so she should make adjustments in her living patterns to avoid worry, strain, anger, or anxiety.

In bottle-fed infants with recurrent indigestion, you will need to study your baby's dietary history to determine what food or other cause is at fault. Meanwhile, if the symptoms are severe, discontinue all feedings for twenty-four hours, giving only arrowroot, barley, or rice water with blackstrap molasses every hour, moving on to increased feedings as tolerated. If *underfeeding* is the source of the problem, begin by feeding skimmed lactic-acid milk with blackstrap molasses in small amounts, every four hours, gradually concentrating the formula until feedings consist of whole lactic-acid milk with added carbohydrate in the form of blackstrap molasses, for a total of 100 cal/lb of body weight, increasing the volume of feedings after the digestive problem subsides. Once your infant has reached the proper weight for age and build, you may switch to a regular cow's-milk mixture, replacing one feeding per day until normal feedings have been completely resumed. If *overfeeding* of one or more of the nutrients is to blame, either as an unbalanced diet or as overall excessive intake, your child may have developed a reduced digestive capacity. All foods should be discontinued and a simple cow's-milk mixture given every four hours, half the amount usually given to infants of your child's age. Between feedings give fluids—arrowroot, barley, or rice water with blackstrap molasses—then increase the volume of feedings until the normal amount is being taken. Finally, add solid foods and vitamin supplements as indicated. *Food intolerances* to allergenic protein or to excessive fat or carbohydrate are another possible cause of the chronic indigestion. If your baby is hypersensitive to cow's-milk protein, switch to evaporated goat's milk or soy milk, adding nonallergenic foods as tolerated. If the problem has been brought on by *excessive fat*, give your infant a formula of skim milk or skimmed lactic-acid milk with blackstrap molasses. If *excessive sugar* in the formula was producing the problem, then give a formula of lactic-acid milk, reinforced with blackstrap molasses as tolerated.

For older children with chronic intestinal indigestion, it is helpful to rely on the foods your child has been able to digest in the past. Remember that the indigestible residues in foods such as milk curd, some fruits and vegetables, and coarse cereals may make the condition worse, and so *low-residue foods are best tolerated* (see Table 15, page 179). If your child is suspected to be *allergic* to certain foods, a series of skin tests may help to determine those that she tolerates well. These may be gradually added until a complete diet is attained. If intestinal putrefaction is noticeable (putrid, offensive stools), restrict your child's protein intake to a minimum, giving readily assimilable carbohydrates free of cellulose (see

Table 19, page 189); the diet might consist of kefir or acidophilus milk with added blackstrap molasses, thin gruel, barley, tapioca, rice, toast or Zweiback, and strained fruit juice. If intestinal fermentation is predominant (sour, frothy stools), then a high-protein diet is called for—meat, chicken or fish, cottage cheese, acidophilus milk or kefir, egg yolk, gelatin—gradually adding cellulose-free starches such as cornstarch, arrowroot, or tapioca one at a time. If your child is *intolerant of fat,* give a high-carbohydrate diet with skim milk, lean meat, fruits, and vegetables.

Table 26 lists some foods that are easy to digest.

TABLE 26
Readily Digestible Foods*

Cereals and Breads	Vegetables (cooked)	Fruits
Cooked cereals	Potatoes	Fruit juices
Stale bread	Carrots	Apples, cooked
	String beans	Pears, "
Dairy Products	Peas	Peaches, "
Milk	Spinach	Bananas, "
Cottage cheese	Beets	Apricots, "
Eggs	Asparagus	Prunes, "
	Cauliflower	
Meats	Squash	**Desserts**
Beef, lean	Tomatoes	Puddings
Lamb, lean		Gelatin (no artificial color or
Chicken, lean		flavor!)
Liver		Ices, natural
Sweetbreads		
Fish		
Oysters		

*After Kugelmass (1940).

For any type of indigestion it is helpful to modify the balance of the intestinal bacteria by giving acidophilus or other naturally fermented dairy products in large quantities; lactose should be given at the same time if not contraindicated, in order to encourage the growth of beneficial bacteria in the intestinal tract.

Are Antacids Harmless? Before providing some herbal remedies for indigestion, we must consider the safety of commonly used over-the-counter antacid medications.

Long considered nontoxic, the element aluminum has now been shown to be absorbed by the gut. Aluminum hydroxide is widely taken as an antacid and must be considered *unsafe* for all of us, but especially children! Apparently aluminum (from antacids, and other dietary sources, such as sodium silico-aluminate, an additive in common table salt, nondairy creamers, etc.) can lead to "disorders of the brain and parathyroid gland" (*Nutrition Reviews*, Vol. 38, p. 242, 1980).

Herbal Preparations

A mild and soothing herbal tea, safe even for infants, may be made from *chamomile*, ½ teaspoon to 1 cup of freshly boiled water. Cover and steep for 5–10 minutes. Drink warm.

Other herbs useful in indigestion, to be used singly, include the following:

Angelica
    (herb or seeds)
or *Dandelion* (leaves)
or *Holy Thistle*
or *Peppermint*
or *Star Anise*
or *Virginia Snakeroot*

Place ½ teaspoon of selected herb in a pot. Add 1 cup freshly boiled water. Cover and steep for 5–10 minutes. Drink warm.

or *Angelica* (root)
or *Dandelion* (root)
or *Ginger*
or *Yellow Gentian*
   (root)

Add ½ teaspoon of selected herb to 1½ pints boiling water. Cover and continue boiling at a slow boil for about 30 minutes. Allow to cool slowly in the closed container. Drink cold, one swallow or 1 tablespoon at a time.

INFECTIOUS DISEASES
See FEVER

IRRITABLE COLON

This disorder is most likely to occur in children with allergic or nervous tendencies, who develop an intolerance to fat or carbohydrates, often during an infectious disease. It is marked by the passage of large quantities of nonbloody mucus in the stools. Either constipation or diarrhea, or both, may be present. An attack may be brought on by the eating of excessive fat or carbohydrate, and is aggravated by a high-residue diet or purgatives.

Diet

Medication is of little help in treating this condition, and dietary regulation is the treatment of choice. With the onset of an attack, *while your doctor is looking for and treating any underlying infection,* it is advisable to give nothing by mouth but fruit juices or barley, rice, or arrowroot water, with added blackstrap molasses, every hour for about twelve hours. Feeding may then be resumed in the form of a bland, nonirritating diet of skimmed, evaporated, powdered, or fermented milk, cooked refined cereals, boiled meat and poultry, and white potato. Avoid raw fruits and vegetables. With improvement in the stools, you may cautiously add strained green vegetables and stewed fruits, and finally eggs, cream, and butter.

Once the acute attack has subsided, *your doctor will evaluate your child to determine what changes need to be made to prevent recurrences.* In order to improve your child's nutritional status, keep him on a bland diet consisting of yogurt or lactic-acid milk, cooked refined cereals, scraped raw apple and ripe banana, tender meats, plain gelatin, pureed vegetables, crackers, toast, or rolls and butter. The diet should be carefully regulated to avoid constipation. (A dose of castor oil is sometimes given at the beginning of treatment to control the accumulation of mucus.)

Herbal Preparations

For their beneficial effect on disorders of the colon, use either of the following herbs:

Blackberry or *Red Raspberry*	If the *leaves* are used, place ½ teaspoon in a pot. Add 1 cup freshly boiled water. Cover and steep for 5–10 minutes. Drink warm. If the *root bark* is used, add ½ teaspoon to 1½ pints of boiling water. Cover and continue boiling at a slow boil for about 30 minutes. Allow to cool slowly in the closed container. Drink cold, one swallow or 1 tablespoon at a time.

To combat constipation, add *senna* leaves to fruit before cooking, and give plenty of fluids between meals. You may also make an herbal tea of *senna,* ½ teaspoon, steeped in 1 cup of freshly boiled water in a covered container for ½ hour. Drink warm or cool, one swallow or 1 tablespoon at a time.

MEASLES

This highly contagious viral disease has come under considerable control in recent years through the use of measles vaccine to confer immunity during infancy or early childhood. However, some children have not received measles immunization and so the disease will continue to appear. Measles begins with symptoms that look like a cold, with a rising fever, following by a rash on about the fourth day. *Your doctor will confirm the diagnosis and follow the course of the illness to make sure there are no dangerous complications.*

(Measles [rubeola] is not to be confused with German measles, or rubella. German measles is a much milder illness in children, and less contagious. The greatest danger of German measles is to pregnant women in whom it may produce abortion, or lead to stillbirth or birth defects in the baby.)

As with other viral disorders, your child should be given the vitamin-C tonic described on page 147, along with the usual supplement formula.

Diet

During fever your child may have very little appetite. Try giving a soft diet of bland foods (see Table 25, page 227) that will not irritate the inflamed throat, fruit juices with added blackstrap molasses, and lots of fluid to encourage elimination of toxins through the kidneys. Rinsing your child's mouth regularly will increase the palatability of food and fluids. The bowel should be kept open. Don't give up on feedings if your child vomits during the early stages of the illness; usually if food is given again a few minutes after vomiting, it will be kept down. Adapt foods to your child's tolerance during the early stage of the disease; you may find she can retain skim milk with added lime water, or whole milk thickened with barley flour. Acid fruit juices may be kept down better than other fluids; if not, try easily digestible semisolid foods such as thick soups, custard, plain gelatin flavored with fruit juice, ice cream, thick purees, or gruels. Diarrhea may be helped with boiled skim milk or acid milk or fermented dairy products.

Herbal Preparations

A gently soothing herbal tea, suitable for infants as well as for older children, may be made from *chamomile*, using ½ teaspoon of the herb to 1 cup of freshly boiled water. Steep, covered, for 5–10 minutes. Drink warm.

A traditional remedy for eruptive diseases such as measles is made from *yarrow*, ¼ ounce to 1 pint of water. Cover and steep for 5–10 minutes. Drink warm.

MIGRAINE, ALLERGIC

Migraine attacks may appear suddenly in older children with no previous similar problems. They consist of periodic attacks of headache, often accompanied or preceded by visual disturbances, and may go on to nausea, vomiting, and finally quiet sleep. Heredity appears to play a role in many cases. One possible cause of migraine is food allergy, the most common culprits being milk, egg, wheat, fish, chocolate, meats, and nuts. If your child is allergy-prone, then food allergy should be strongly suspected. *Your doctor will supervise the treatment,* which will include quiet, darkened surroundings, with avoidance of emotional excitement, and possibly medication.

Diet

All foods should be withheld initially except for non-allergenic fruit juices and herbal teas, with blackstrap molasses. To prevent recurrent attacks, it will be necessary to eliminate allergenic foods from your child's diet, beginning with any foods that have produced a reaction on skin-testing. If this doesn't help the problem or if skin tests don't indicate any offending foods, then an elimination diet should be begun, starting with a soft elimination diet (see Table 12, page 159) and gradually adding presumably nonallergenic foods until an adequate nutrient intake is reached. If such a nonallergenic diet still fails to help, then your child may, *under your doctor's supervision*, be put on a so-called ketogenic diet (high in fats, moderate in proteins, and low in carbohydrates), containing no foods to which your child is sensitive, and foods low in salt and total fluids. Such a diet produces mild tissue dehydration, which often helps to reduce allergic reactivity. Of course, emotional and physical disturbances should also be avoided, to help prevent future attacks.

Herbal Preparations

Use any of the following for relief of headache:

Balm or *Lavender* or *Gotu kola*	Place ½ teaspoon of selected herb in a pot. Add 1 cup freshly boiled water. Cover and steep for 5–10 minutes. Drink warm, one mouthful or 1 tablespoon at a time.

See also: ALLERGY

MILK INTOLERANCE

We have stated earlier that human milk is the perfect food for developing infants. This is true. Milk does contain just about all the nutrients required by growing infants, including all the vitamins and minerals, except for vitamin D, which the body can manufacture with only a few minutes in the sun.

Lactase Insufficiency. Now, it is a relatively unusual condition, but some infants do not have an adequate amount of the enzyme lactase, and an insufficiency of this enzyme may explain gastrointestinal problems in an infant such as constant diarrhea and gas.

Lactose, or milk sugar, is a disaccharide that must be broken down, or hydrolyzed, into glucose and galactose by the enzyme lactase. In cases where this enzyme is insufficient or missing entirely, unabsorbed milk sugar stays inside the lumen of the intestine, retaining water and causing bloating and cramping, as well as the other symptoms.

Technically speaking, this problem is not an allergy to milk but rather the result of an insufficiency of an enzyme. There are people, however, who are allergic to milk and all dairy products; but if your child, you yourself, or any member of your family exhibits the symptoms described earlier after ingesting milk or dairy products, it would be advisable to experiment and see if you can tolerate a small amount of dairy. You may be among the approximately 30 million adults in the United States who have very little lactase, and although they can consume small quantities of milk or dairy, they are unable to eat large servings of ice cream, cheese, milk, or other milk products without experiencing the symptoms that are caused by undigested lactose. There is an ethnic factor here, because lactase deficiency is found particularly among Eastern European Jewish people, American Indians, Orientals, and adult black people.

Milk Allergy. For those who are suspected to have a true allergy to cow's milk—that is, to the protein in milk and dairy products—we must evaluate the allergy and then devise alternatives to milk formulas for the infant and alternative calcium sources for older children and adults.

A true milk-protein allergy is quite a rare phenomenon, appearing in only about 1 percent of the infant population. If your infant is receiving a milk-based formula and exhibits classic allergic symptoms such as wheezing, eczematous rash, or runny nose, you should suspect a milk protein allergy.

Diet

If you do suspect an allergy to milk protein, switch the formula to one based on predigested protein; then *your pediatrician will probably test your infant's stool for secondary lactose intolerance.* After several months on a hypoallergenic formula, milk will be tried again. If your baby is still hypersensitive to the milk, you will periodically try to see if she can tolerate it.

Distinguishing Allergy from Lactose Intolerance. It is not easy to differentiate clinically between the often identical symptoms of milk-protein allergy and lactose intolerance, but there are some simple office tests that have been devised for this purpose. In one procedure a fresh stool sample is tested for its pH level and to see if glucose is present. An acidic stool is a good diagnostic indicator of lactose intolerance, and is the result of the bacterial breakdown of lactose within the colon. In this test a urine dipstick for determining pH is inserted into a stool sample; after a moment it is removed, washed off, and checked for acidity. While the normal pH is 7 to 8, it will drop to about 5.5 in cases of lactose intolerance. The stool is then tested for the presence of glucose, which will appear when small amounts of lactose are hydrolyzed within the colon but not absorbed. Using a glucose indicator, again a dipstick, your pediatrician will check for a reading of 1+ or higher, which would indicate lactose intolerance. If both these tests are negative for your infant, then it is unlikely that she is suffering from lactase insufficiency. In this case, a true allergy to milk proteins is highly likely.

Remember this: milk-protein allergy usually will appear within the first two months of life, sometimes within the first ten days, and then usually disappears between ages one and four, as the tolerance to milk protein increases. Even the traditional soy-based formula for allergic infants will sometimes cause a different type of protein reaction. In this case you may have to use a formula containing predigested protein to avoid reaction. It is important that we emphasize again that people who avoid milk or dairy products for any reason must be receiving supplementary calcium if they want to avoid calcium deficiency. In addition, a vitamin-D supplement is also required.

If you suspect a lactose problem or a milk-protein allergy, you must learn to read labels carefully for lactose content. Remember, though, that not all milk products have the same effect. For example, naturally aged cheddar cheese contains very little lactose and is therefore usually well tolerated by the lactase-deficient individual. It is also important to remember that this is not an all-or-nothing situation, because a small amount of even a lactose-rich food can be tolerated by many sensitive individuals.

A few suitable alternatives to regular milk do exist that can be tolerated by many people. These include milk treated with powdered lactase enzyme or sweet acidophilus milk; and partially fermented milk products such as sour cream, cottage cheese, and some other cheeses are often well accepted by lactose-intolerant individuals. Remember, however, that most commercially prepared yogurts have had lactose added to enhance their texture, and lactose is also found very frequently as a filler in many pharmaceutical products.

Which foods contain lactose? Let's begin with the beverages. Here we find all kinds of milk drinks prepared with malted-milk powder, Ovaltine, chocolate drinks, liqueurs, cordials, and even some instant coffees. Meats such as liver, brain, sweetbreads, liverwurst, frankfurters, and cold cuts that have dry milk in them should also be looked at with suspicion. But it is noteworthy that all kosher meat products and foods that are marked "parve" do *not* contain milk. All cheeses contain lactose; the highest amounts are found in low-fat and creamed cottage cheese and ricotta. The lowest lactose content is found in aged natural cheddar cheese, Brie, Camembert, Gruyère, Limburger, Monterey. Bread products containing lactose are simple to keep in mind: any bread, cereal, crackers, pancakes, waffle mix, or French toast made with milk products should be avoided or eaten in only small quantities. Desserts such as milk-based puddings, custards, or cookies, pie crusts, cakes, and pie fillings made with milk should be avoided. Naturally, ice cream is often milk-rich. In addition, you must pay particular attention to a whole variety of other foods that may contain lactose, including yogurt, as previously mentioned, breaded fish, meat and poultry that have been frozen; packaged mixes, molasses, butterscotch, chocolate candy, caramels; cream sauces and gravies; and diabetic products, to name just a few.

For those of you who make your own yogurt, you can reduce the lactose content by allowing fermentation to run longer than the usual time. This will yield a low-lactose product that is still rich in calcium. Other good sources of calcium are canned sardines and salmon that have the bones, green leafy vegetables, dried beans, and some nuts. If you are not getting a sufficient amount of calcium from your foods owing to a lactose intolerance or a milk-protein allergy, you may want to take supplementary calcium, and again let us emphasize vitamin D for children who are growing, to prevent the development of rickets.

You can also buy the enzyme lactase commercially today without a prescription. It is known as Lact-Aid or Lact-o-Zyme, and comes in a liquid or powdered form. It can be added to whole milk, skim, fresh, reconstituted, canned, or dry milk, cream, or infant formula, and will convert lactose to glucose and galactose. When you use the liquid form, all you need to do is add 4 to 5 drops to a quart of milk, shake or mix the milk, and then refrigerate it for twenty-four hours, during which time the lactose is hydrolyzed. This treated milk can then be used as it is or for cooking, making cheese, yogurt, baking, or in any other way that regular milk is used. One note of caution, however: the sugars in this product are more rapidly absorbed and are *not for diabetics!*

Herbal Preparations

For indigestion associated with milk intolerance, any one of the following herbs may be used to prepare a gently soothing herbal tea for children of all ages, including infants:

Chamomile or *Anise* or *Fennel*	Place ½ teaspoon of selected herb in a pot. Add 1 cup freshly boiled water. Cover and steep for 5–10 minutes. Drink warm. (A *hibiscus* leaf may be added to any of these herbs for flavoring.)

MONONUCLEOSIS

This infectious disease is common among children and young adults. It is usually marked by an elevated temperature and swelling of the lymph glands, especially about the neck. Your doctor will be able to confirm the diagnosis through appropriate tests. Although this disorder is not generally serious in itself, it may last for weeks, and so it is important to maintain good nutrition to help protect against complications. As with other viral diseases, vitamin C, in the form of the "cocktail" described on page 147, should be helpful.

Diet

During the acute stage of the disease, your child should receive a bland soft diet with plenty of fluids between feedings. (See Table 25, page 227, and Table 23, page 209.) Food and drink will be more appealing if you are careful to encourage frequent cleansing of the nose and rinsing of the mouth and throat. If whole milk is not well tolerated, try fermented or acidified skim milk with blackstrap molasses. If there is diarrhea, you may give raw grated apple pulp between feedings. It is very important to maintain frequent fluid intake to guard against dehydration; *if your child won't take enough fluids orally, your doctor may need to give them by other means.*

As the acute infection subsides, you may begin to add semisolid foods that are not irritating to the mucous membranes. Anemia may develop during the course of the disease, requiring additional iron in the form of supplements or iron-rich foods.

Herbal Preparations

Agar-agar may be added to cereals, soups, or other foods, to soothe irritated mucous membranes and absorb toxins. Start with approximately ¼ gram and increase as indicated.

Any of the following herbs may be used to make a soothing herbal tea:

Mullein or *Plantain*	Place ½ teaspoon of selected herb in a pot. Add 1 cup freshly boiled water. Cover and steep for 5–10 minutes. Drink warm.
or *Sweet Fern*	Add ½ teaspoon of root to 1½ pints boiling water. Cover and continue boiling at a slow boil for about 30 minutes. Allow to cool slowly in the closed container. Drink cold, one swallow or 1 tablespoon at a time.

A soothing and refreshing gargle may be made from *spearmint,* ½ teaspoon steeped for 5–10 minutes in 1 cup of freshly boiled water. Allow to cool before using as a gargle.

MULTIPLE SCLEROSIS

This distressing disease, which sometimes strikes teenagers and for which there is no "acceptable" treatment, seems to be ameliorated to some degree by evening primrose oil, as reported by Dr. D. F. Horrobin in *Medical Hypotheses,* Vol. 5, pp. 365–378 (1979):

"Multiple Sclerosis: The Rational Basis for Treatment with Colchicine and Evening Primrose Oil.

Abstract:

Multiple sclerosis (MS) is a disease with no known treatment. In view of this and of its distressing nature patients are attracted by any new concepts. As a reaction to this neurologists are sometimes excessively sceptical and fail to consider new approaches seriously. Recent attempts have been made to treat multiple sclerosis with polyunsaturated fatty acids and with colchicine. This approach is not arbitrary and is firmly grounded in fundamental basic scientific concepts. In patients with multiple sclerosis there is evidence of both an abnormality in essential fatty acid metabolism and an abnormality in lymphocyte function. It is now apparent that the fatty acid abnormality may cause the lymphocyte abnormality and that both may be improved by dietary manipulation. There is also evidence that the demyelination may be associated with recurrent inflammatory episodes and with entry of calcium into the cytoplasm. In vitro colchicine has been shown to have actions compatible with regulation of cytoplasmic calcium and in two diseases characterised by intermittent inflammatory episodes (Behçet's syndrome and familial Mediterranean fever) it has been found to prevent or to reduce the severity of such episodes.

Preliminary results suggest the combined therapy with evening primrose oil and colchicine may be of considerable value.*

Diet

Use of Evening Primrose Oil as a Food

Since 1930 it has been known that certain polyunsaturated fatty acids cannot be synthesized by the body and must be provided in the diet. It is now known that these essential fatty acids (EFAs) are of two main series, those derived from linoleic acid and those derived from α-linoleic acid. This report concerns the linoleic acid series.

The US Recommended Dietary Allowances suggests that a minimum of 1% of the total calorie intake should be in the form of EFAs. However the recent report from the FAO suggested that the minimum intake in adults should be revised up to 3% and that in pregnancy 4.5% might be required. In lactation it was proposed that 5–7% of the total calorie intake should be in the form of EFAs. Requirements in infants and growing children may be similar to those in pregnancy and lactation.

In most Western diets the major part of food EFAs is in the form of linoleic acid (LA). There are much smaller amounts of arachidonic acid (AA), particularly in meat and seaweed, and very small amounts of gamma-linolenic acid (GLA) and dihomogammalinolenic acid (DGLA). Linoleic acid is converted to GLA, GLA to DGLA, DGLA to AA and AA on to longer chain acids.

Until relatively recently the relative functions of these various compounds were not understood. It was known that LA was converted through to AA and beyond but not how effective LA itself might be in combating EFA deficiency. A recent observation in cats

*While quantities for primrose oil usage are not given, this novel approach is included for consideration of those afflicted, to be discussed with their physicians.

has however demonstrated that linoleic acid itself is almost completely inert as an EFA. It must be converted to GLA and then onwards in order to be effective.

Cats lack the enzymes necessary for conversion of LA to GLA and of DGLA to AA. They therefore provide a unique opportunity for the study of EFA deficiency. In cats fed an EFA deficient diet there was no difference between animals which were and were not supplemented with safflower oil, an oil very rich in linoleic acid (about 73% by weight). Safflower oil is the most potent commonly available source of EFAs. Whether or not the animals were given safflower oil they were all equally ill showing growth failure, apathetic behavior, dry scaling coats with severe dandruff, skin ulceration, defective wound healing, susceptibility to infection, underdeveloped testes in males and absence of estrous cycles in females. When safflower oil was half replaced by evening primrose oil, a change which did not alter substantially the LA intake but did provide 2.9% of total fatty acids in the diet as GLA, a dramatic change took place in the animals. Within 10 days coat and skin condition substantially improved and wound healing became normal. Estrous cycles returned but growth and appetite did not alter. The group provided evidence that the cat, as well as being unable to convert LA to GLA also cannot convert DGLA to AA.

Summary:
Multiple sclerosis (MS) is one of the most distressing of all diseases. There are no accepted methods of treating it even though many different proposals have been made. Understandably, patients with MS, who are often highly intelligent, take a great interest in ongoing research and are eager to try any new approaches. Because such approaches have so regularly proved disappointing, neurologists tend to become blasé about new ideas, to fail to investigate them thoroughly and to take an unduly negative attitude.

The uses of polyunsaturated fats and of colchicine

have recently been proposed in MS. These are not arbitrary proposals but have a firm basis in what is known about the disease and in sound experimental laboratory science.

Herbal Preparations

For sleeplessness, use *passionflower*, ¼ to ½ teaspoon of the herb to 1 cup freshly boiled water. Cover and steep for 5–10 minutes. Drink warm.

MUMPS

Your doctor will need to determine whether swollen glands around the neck or ear represent mumps or some other condition. The symptoms of painful, swollen salivary glands take two or three weeks to develop after exposure to mumps. The swelling may last up to ten days, although it will go away sooner in mild cases.

Diet

A soft diet of bland foods (see Table 25, page 227) is best during the acute stages of the illness. If there is pain on chewing, your child will have less trouble with semisolid foods such as thin cereal gruels, soups, ice cream, custard, or liquids taken through a straw. If citrus juices are irritating to the inflamed glands, try the cooked juices of bland fruits, perhaps with added blackstrap molasses to increase energy content. A mild alkaline solution, such as bicarbonate of soda, may be used to cleanse your child's mouth and relieve uncomfortable dryness; this may also help encourage better food and fluid intake. As temperature returns to normal, you can begin adding other foods to the diet according to tolerance. Anemia may be present, which will be helped by extra iron supplements, if your child is not sensitive to them.

Herbal Preparations

For a soothing gargle, place ½ teaspoon of *spearmint* in a pot. Add 1 cup freshly boiled water. Cover and steep for 5–10 minutes, then strain and cool for use as a mouthwash or gargle.

The following herbs, used singly, will help to stimulate your child's appetite:

Holy Thistle:	Place ½ teaspoon of herb in a pot. Add one cup freshly boiled water. Cover and steep for 5–10 minutes. Drink warm.
or *Yellow Gentian Root* or *Sweet Fern Root*	Add ½ teaspoon of selected herb to 1½ pints of boiling water. Cover and continue boiling at a slow boil for about 30 minutes. Allow to cool slowly in the closed container. Drink cold, one swallow or 1 tablespoon at a time.

As a pain reliever, place ½ teaspoon of *passionflower* in a pot. Add one cup of freshly boiled water. Cover and steep for 5–10 minutes. Drink warm.

NAUSEA
See REGURGITATION, NAUSEA, AND VOMITING

NOSE, RUNNING
See COLDS; HAY FEVER

OTITIS MEDIA

Middle-ear infections are quite common in youngsters, and can be quite painful with earache and often impaired hearing. Well-nourished children will often recover spontaneously from otitis media, but a poorly nourished child will need to be treated not only for the ear problem but also to improve his resistance to future infection. *Your doctor will help investigate the cause of the problem and may prescribe medication to prevent complications.* Allergy is a possible cause of otitis media, and so you may need to review your child's diet to see if a sensitivity to cow's milk or other food might have brought on the attack. If allergy is suspected, follow the procedures suggested in the "Allergy" section.

Diet

During the acute stage of the infection, limit food to what your child can tolerate, being sure to give plenty of fluids to prevent dehydration. Sucking may be painful for infants, and so you may need to adapt feeding techniques to give your baby enough fluids. As the infection clears up, your child's ability to digest foods will improve, and you will be able to begin correcting his nutritional status, gradually increasing dietary intake until you are giving concentrated feedings that are high in alkaline-forming fruits and vegetables (see Table 16, page 184), and moderate in protein, along with supplementary vitamins. Your pediatrician may recommend extra supplements in addition to the usual "Longevity Formula" (see Appendix B).

Herbal Preparations

For earache, squeeze *garlic* juice into a little olive oil and apply the oil to a wad of cotton. Insert into ear.

For a calming, pain-relieving tea, place ½ teaspoon of *passionflower* in a pot. Add one cup of freshly boiled water. Cover and steep for 5–10 minutes. Drink warm.

PNEUMONIA

Pneumonia often begins with the symptoms of an upper respiratory infection such as cold or flu. With modern antibiotic therapy it has become possible to treat successfully many formerly life-threatening forms of pneumonia, especially those caused by bacterial organisms. *Your doctor will determine the best treatment in your child's case.* Viral forms of pneumonia will be helped by the vitamin-C tonic described on page 147.

Diet

Dietary regulation, *in conjunction with your doctor's treatment plan,* can speed your child's recovery. In the case of a more acute, short-term form of pneumonia such as lobar pneumonia, your child should be given a liquid diet consisting of small frequent feedings of acid milk or fermented dairy with added blackstrap molasses. Nonfermentable fruit juices, such as grapefruit, pineapple, and lemon, with added blackstrap molasses and a little table salt, should be given hourly between feedings. *Severe cases may require supplementation in the form of intravenous or intramuscular feedings, administered by your doctor.* He may also advise enemas to relieve abdominal swelling.

In prolonged forms of pneumonia in a debilitated child, such as bronchopneumonia, you will need to encourage optimum caloric intake, with moderate protein content in the diet especially after the acute stage, and large quantities of carbohydrate to meet your child's increased energy needs. Fats will tend to produce digestive disturbances and should be kept to a minimum. Plenty of minerals should be provided, both in fruits and vegetables and if necessary in extra supplements as well. Throughout the course of the illness be sure to encourage maximum fluid intake.

Herbal Preparations

An herbal tea for fever and its accompanying inflammatory complaints may be made from either one of the following:

Yarrow or *Eucalyptus*	Place ½ teaspoon of selected herb in a pot. Add 1 cup freshly boiled water. Cover and steep for 5–10 minutes. Drink warm.

An expectorant tea to help clear mucus from the breathing passages may be made from *ephedra,* ½ teaspoon to 1 pint of freshly boiled water. Steep in covered container for 5–10 minutes. Drink warm.

To stimulate a flagging appetite, use any one of the following herbs:

Holy Thistle	Place ½ teaspoon of herb in a pot. Add one cup freshly boiled water. Cover and steep for 5–10 minutes. Drink warm.
or *Yellow Gentian Root* or *Sweet Fern Root*	Add ½ teaspoon of selected herb to 1½ pints of boiling water. Cover and continue boiling at a slow boil for about 30 minutes. Allow to cool slowly in the closed container. Drink cold, one swallow or 1 tablespoon at a time.

PSORIASIS

This skin disease, which is sometimes hereditary, usually comes on slowly and may first appear in later childhood. Today there are a number of complex medical treatments for this often frustrating condition, but regulation of the diet has proven helpful in the past and should not be forgotten as one means of relief.

Diet

A low-protein diet has been most helpful in stubborn or acute cases, with specific limitation of proteins that have been found to aggravate the condition—milk, cheese, eggs, meat, fish, and fowl. While restricting protein intake, however, *your doctor must supervise your child's diet* to make sure that there are adequate levels of protein supplied—approximately 0.7 gram per pound of body weight—to avoid deficiency states. If your child is obese, a low-carbohydrate diet, along with reduction in total calories, may also be helpful; your doctor will need to approve any reduction in food intake to make sure your child's nutritional status will not suffer. In any case, salt, sweets, indigestible or stimulating foods should be eliminated from your child's diet.

Mineral Remedy

A warm, soaking bath in a good natural bath salt from mineral-rich, *unpolluted* sea water (such as Dead Sea salts), given twice a day, is a soothing and healing treatment for eczema.

PYLORIC STENOSIS

This condition, generally occurring in infants during the first ten weeks of life, and most common in boys, consists of an obstruction of the pylorus, or opening of the stomach into the intestine. Symptoms include projectile-vomiting and exaggerated peristaltic contractions. Projectile-vomiting can have a number of causes. *This condition should always be immediately called to the attention of your doctor.*

It has become fairly routine procedure for pyloric stenosis to be treated surgically; however, there is evidence that in many cases the condition will eventually correct itself with medical and nutritional support alone. *With your doctor's approval,* then, you may decide to undertake dietary treatment under his supervision, before resorting to surgery.

Diet

A breast-fed infant may continue to nurse, 5 minutes at a time, at 4-hour intervals. However, thick feedings are generally preferred, since these favor nonperistaltic stomach contractions and hence discourage vomiting. For this purpose, milk may be expressed from the breasts and given with added carbohydrate (such as arrowroot, barley, flour, rice flour), or boiled with cereal. If your baby vomits after these feedings, you may feed him again, twice if necessary.

Bottle-fed infants can be given thick feedings made of evaporated milk, barley, flour, and blackstrap molasses (¼ teaspoon per bottle), or a concentrated formula of half-strength evaporated milk and blackstrap molasses, or whole lactic-acid milk and blackstrap molasses. These are to be given at four-hour intervals in small amounts. If the baby vomits, refeed an equal quantity immediately after vomiting.

With concentrated feedings of low fluid content, as well as with the loss of fluid through vomiting, there is a danger of dehydration, so it is important to supply adequate fluids. Give water in small amounts one hour *before* feedings, but never after. If your baby has difficulty keeping water down during the day, try giving it at night when feedings are over.

Your pediatrician will watch your baby's progress closely. If there is no improvement after a week or two of dietary management, he will likely recommend surgery.

Herbal Preparations

A safe and soothing tea for infants may be made of *chamomile,* ½ teaspoon to 1 cup of freshly boiled water. Cover and steep for 5–10 minutes. Drink warm.

REGURGITATION, NAUSEA, AND VOMITING

There can be many reasons for regurgitation and vomiting in infants and children. These symptoms serve as a defense mechanism, the stomach rejecting food that is unsuitable in quantity or quality, thus protecting the child against its harmful effects. Regurgitation is defined as the incomplete expulsion of material from the stomach, which is usually returned through reswallowing. Vomiting entails the expulsion of all or part of the stomach contents from the mouth, and may be projectile in nature. Nausea is a warning symptom that regurgitation or vomiting is about to occur. Infants have a much greater tendency to vomit than do older children, but *all cases of vomiting, especially in infants, should be called to the attention of your pediatrician,* who will need to determine the cause and prescribe appropriate treatment.

Diet

Many cases of vomiting are related to diet and feeding problems, and simple adjustments in feedings will clear them up. In infants, both breast- and bottle-fed, the trouble may be due to *excessive swallowing of air* during feeding. Air-swallowing may occur because of mechanical problems in feeding, or because the child is not receiving enough food and is gulping air to produce a feeling of fullness. If your child is not receiving enough breast milk, *consult your doctor;* you may need to add supplementary feedings of cow's, goat's, soy, or other milk formula to meet nutritional needs. Bottle-fed infants may be underfed because their formula is too dilute; reevaluation of the formula and a switch to more concentrated feedings may help to clear up the problem.

Too-frequent feedings are another possible cause of vomiting; a mother may nurse her baby every time he cries, when in fact he may be crying because he has indigestion rather than because he is hungry. Regular nursing at four-hour intervals is the solution here. The infant may be receiving *too much food,* gulping down breast milk or receiving large volumes of formula in the bottle. Limiting breast-feeding to one breast at a time for 5 minutes, every 4 hours, and bottle-feeding to fairly concentrated mixtures will help control vomiting under these circumstances.

Infants may be vomiting because of *allergies* to substances in breast milk or formula. Nursing mothers must review their diet to see what they have eaten to which their baby might be sensitive, and should eliminate the common allergenic foods such as egg, wheat, and chocolate from their diet. Or the mother may switch to a simple diet of boiled milk or yogurt, fruits, and vegetables, adding new foods one at a time and noting the baby's reaction. Bottle-fed infants may vomit because of an allergy to cow's milk, in which case you can switch to evaporated milk, goat's milk, or soy milk. Orange juice may also produce vomiting; try switching to other juices such as pineapple or grapefruit, to see if they are tolerated. Older children also may have nausea and vomiting from food allergy. They may refuse certain foods out of an instinctive desire to protect themselves against allergic reaction, and when these foods are forced on them, they vomit as a defense mechanism. Pay attention to your child's likes and dislikes; they are often indications of hypersensitivities to particular foods.

Bottle-fed babies may have problems with *indigestible protein curds* from cow's milk; switching to an evaporated, acid, fermented, or powdered milk may help. Breast-fed infants don't have problems with the protein curd in human milk; nor are they intolerant of the natural sugar in human milk. But bottle-fed babies may develop vomiting from *excessive sugar* added to their formula. If sugar content has recently been increased, or if it is over 15 percent, the formula may require adjustment. *Too much fat* in the diet may also cause vomiting. If breast-fed babies nurse for long periods they will receive the fat-rich last portions of the breast milk. Reducing their nursing time to less than 5 minutes will provide the fore milk which is less rich in fat; feed every 4 hours, and gradually lengthen feedings to about 8 minutes. Vomiting may occur in many *infectious diseases* as a result of digestive disturbances. Once the disease has been diagnosed, feed your child the diet appropriate to the particular illness.

Until your doctor has helped to determine the reason for vomiting, don't force food on your child. Until medical help arrives, allow your child's digestive system to have a rest, giving small quantities of water only as tolerated, cautiously increasing the quantity or adding a little fruit juice. Be guided by your child's wants; if she asks for solid food, try a cracker or a small amount of unsweetened applesauce. If vomiting occurs again, wait a couple of hours before giving more food or fluids, and then give a very small quantity of water or cracked ice, cautiously increasing the quantity as tolerated at intervals thereafter.

Herbal Preparations

A good remedy for vomiting is *red raspberry*. Use ½ teaspoon of the *leaf* to a cup of freshly boiled water. Cover and steep for 5–10 minutes. Drink warm. If you use the *root bark*, add ½ teaspoon to 1½ pints of boiling water. Cover and continue boiling at a slow boil for about 30 minutes. Allow to cool slowly in the closed container. Drink cold, one swallow or 1 tablespoon at a time.

For a soothing herbal tea, used widely for infants, use any one of the following herbs:

Chamomile
or *Anise Seeds*
or *Fennel*

Place ½ teaspoon of selected herb in a pot. Add 1 cup freshly boiled water. Steep for 5–10 minutes. Drink warm. (May be flavored while steeping with one *hibiscus* leaf.)

RHEUMATIC FEVER

This disorder may have extremely variable symptoms, involving the joints, the heart, and other parts of the body. It often begins with a streptococcus infection in the throat, and the first attack commonly occurs in children between the ages of four and eighteen. Rheumatic fever can cause permanent damage to the heart valves, and so *it is important to consult your pediatrician* when strep throat is suspected, so that it can be cleared up with appropriate medical treatment.

Diet

The dietary strategy is aimed at maintaining optimal nutritional status during the course of the acute attack, to minimize the risk of cardiac damage. Your child should receive a soft diet consisting of easily digestible foods (see Table 26, page 232), with large quantities of fluids to help the elimination of toxic substances and to replace water lost through sweating. As the acute symptoms are alleviated, begin as soon as possible to make gradual additions of easily assimilable foods to maintain a high caloric intake. If your child resists feeding, make extra efforts to provide food that appeals to his palate. Anemia may develop in the course of the illness, and will be helped with green vegetables, liver, and iron supplements if necessary.

Herbal Preparations

For *sore throat,* see the herbs listed under "Sore Throat."

For *fever,* see herbs listed under "Fever."

Witch-hazel extract not only makes a good gargle for relief of sore throat but may also be applied externally for *joint pains,* which sometimes accompany rheumatic fever.

SINUSITIS

Chronic infection of the sinus cavities in the bones about the nose may be accompanied by headache, facial pain, and sometimes postnasal drip. *Your doctor will need to investigate* chronic sinus problems carefully in order to see if they have been brought on by allergy or by nutritional deficiencies. Symptomatic relief of stuffiness before feedings will encourage your child to take more food; the herbal vaporizer mix, which can only be used in suitable hot-water vaporizers described below will be useful in this regard.

Diet

Until the cause of the problem has been determined, maintain your child on a balanced diet, supplemented with the usual vitamin/mineral formula (see Appendix B) to enhance his resistance to infection. The problem may be further helped by limiting his intake of salt, sugar, and water to induce mild tissue dehydration.

If allergy is found to be an underlying factor in your child's sinusitis, your doctor will help you to determine which foods or other substances are bringing on the allergic reaction, and your child's diet will reflect these findings (see "Allergy").

Herbal Preparations

Use vaporizer at night to relieve congestion. The herbal mix consists of ½ ounce each of *boneset, burdock,* and *eucalyptus.* Place herbs in a cheesecloth bag and boil for 20 minutes in 2 quarts of water. Strain. Place in vaporizer, then dilute with water to reach proper level.

SORE THROAT

A sore throat is often the first sign of a cold or other infectious disease. Of course, it is better to err on the side of caution in the case of childhood illnesses, and so if this is your first baby, *you shouldn't be reluctant to ask your doctor to take a look at your child whenever sore throat occurs,* especially if there is a fever, since treatment may vary depending on the nature of the infection. Tonsillitis, for example, is one possible diagnosis. More experienced mothers will generally give their child a day or two to get better at home with plenty of vitamin C (see the vitamin-C tonic on page 147), rest, and keeping warm, with lots of liquids and soft diet as described below. Then, if the condition gets worse or doesn't improve, the pediatrician will be consulted on the third day. (*Sore throat accompanied by fever and convulsions is* never *for home treatment, and your child should be taken to the hospital if this combination of symptoms appears.*)

Diet

In order to minimize irritation of the throat tissues, stick with bland liquid diets for breast-fed or bottle-fed infants. For breast-fed infants the duration of nursing should be decreased and solid feedings eliminated or decreased, with bland fruit juices given between feedings. Bottle-fed infants should have their milk diluted or the amount of formula decreased, with solid feedings discontinued and fruit juice given between feedings. Older children may be fed cooked cereal, stewed fruit and skim milk, with fruit juices between meals.

If your child develops a fever, follow the usual procedure of cutting total food intake in half to prevent digestive disturbances (see "Fever"), especially in infants. If your child refuses to eat or drink and is getting dehydrated, your doctor may need to give fluids by artificial means.

Herbal Preparations

For a soothing gargle, use *witch-hazel* extract. *Acacia gum* is another soothing remedy for sore throat. Suck on a piece of the dried gum. The following herbs, used singly, may be used to prepare teas to relieve sore throat.

Horehound or *Mullein*	Place ½ teaspoon of selected herb in a pot. Add 1 cup freshly boiled water. Cover and steep for 5–10 minutes. Drink warm.
Licorice or *Marshmallow** or *Goldenseal** or *Slippery Elm*	Add ½ teaspoon of selected herb to 1½ pints boiling water. Cover and continue boiling at a slow boil for about 30 minutes. Allow to cool slowly in the closed container. Drink cold, one swallow or 1 tablespoon at a time.

THYROID DISORDERS

Thyroid-deficiency states include *goiter*, a swelling of the thyroid gland owing to low iodine intake, and *hypothyroidism*, an underactivity of the thyroid gland resulting in retarded growth and development. *Your doctor will determine the diagnosis and may prescribe thyroid-hormone replacement.*

Diet

In these conditions, there is impairment of the body's ability to absorb food from the digestive tract and to utilize it efficiently, and so the hypothyroid child will require more nutrients for his body weight than a normal

*May be used as a gargle as well as drunk as a tea.

child. A hypothyroid child may appear heavy for his age and build; some parents might mistake this for a sign of overfeeding and try reducing his nutrient intake. Actually, it is very important to insure a proper, carefully balanced diet in these cases; adequate supplies of necessary nutrients can help greatly in correcting many cases of hypothyroidism. Associated digestive problems such as vomiting, diarrhea, or gastric distress may be helped by giving a digestive enzyme before meals.

Herbal Preparations

Kelp tablets (no sugar or artificial flavors, binders, etc.!) often help to stimulate thyroid function.

An herbal tea to stimulate the thyroid is made of *Oregon grape root,* ½ teaspoon of the granulated root to 1½ pints of freshly boiled water. Cover and steep for 30 minutes. Strain. Take one swallow or 1 tablespoon at a time. Inform your physician if you use this preparation so that he can adjust thyroid hormone dosage.

Hyperthyroidism. Here, exactly the opposite reaction occurs. The excessive production of thyroid hormone leads to a speeding up of the body's metabolic rate, with symptoms such as nervousness, overactivity, and weight loss often despite increased appetite. *Your doctor will determine the proper treatment for this condition,* but in the meantime it is important to provide your child with emotional and physical rest, a high-calorie diet, lots of fluids, and adequate iodine.

Diet

Because your child's body is burning up food at an increased rate, it is very important to provide a diet high in calories. This may require some ingenuity, since if the diet is too bulky, he may feel full before enough nutrients have been consumed. Protein and carbohydrate intake should be high, to help replace the rapidly broken down tissues and to prevent further tissue loss. Fluids should be given in large quantities, especially when there is fluid loss through elevation of temperature, profuse sweating, diarrhea, or vomiting. (*If your child can't take enough fluids by mouth, your doctor may need to give additional amounts by other means.*)

Herbal Preparations

For a calming effect on your child's overstimulated system, prepare an herbal tea of one of the following:

Chamomile or *Passionflower*	Place ½ teaspoon of selected herb in a pot. Add 1 cup freshly boiled water. Cover and steep for 5–10 minutes. Drink warm.

TONSILLITIS

This common childhood complaint, characterized by swollen, red tonsils (and often adenoids as well), is usually caused by streptococcus bacteria or by a virus. In the past, tonsillectomy was done fairly routinely in children with recurrent problems with tonsillitis, or even at its first appearance. However, this disorder tends to correct itself with proper nutritional and medical support, and the trend today is away from surgery. After all, the tonsils and adenoids are important protective structures guarding one of the main entrances to your child's body, and they should not be removed unless there is a serious obstruction of breathing or other complications. *Your doctor should follow any case of tonsillitis,* and in severe cases may recommend tonsillectomy.

Diet

Feeding may be difficult because of pain on swallowing. Don't force your infant to take more food than he can tolerate, or digestive problems may develop. For older children a soft diet of thin cereal, strained fruit, cold natural jellies, and skim milk may be given, with cooked fruit juices between meals. Avoid all coarse or irritating foods or fluids.

If tonsillectomy is performed, your child will receive only bland fluids the first day after surgery, adding soft, nonirritating foods as tolerance is regained. After the second day, postsurgery children usually don't have trouble swallowing, and a normal diet can be gradually resumed. Remember that hospital diets are not always wisely designed; don't let your child be loaded up with sweets or overly refined foods that you would avoid at home. Feed with care and simplicity, especially those recipes from Book IV that have been favored.

Herbal Preparations

For a soothing gargle, use *witch-hazel* extract.

A piece of *acacia gum* may also be sucked for relief of sore throat.

Any one of the following herbs may be used to prepare a tea to relieve sore throat.

Horehound or *Mullein*	Place ½ teaspoon of selected herb in a pot. Add 1 cup freshly boiled water. Cover and steep for 5–10 minutes. Drink warm.
Licorice or *Marshmallow** or *Goldenseal** or *Slippery Elm*	Add ½ teaspoon of selected herb to 1½ pints boiling water. Cover and continue boiling at a slow boil for about 30 minutes. Allow to cool slowly in the closed container. Drink cold, one swallow or 1 tablespoon at a time.

---

* May be used as a gargle as well as drunk as a tea.

TOOTH DECAY

As in other illnesses and disorders discussed in this section, the digestive system is of prime importance in the development of tooth decay. Recent research, as reported by Dr. Michael Cole, of the National Institutes of Health, in the Washington *Post,* has shown that "the antibodies for all these mucous membranes are formed in the intestines. As they develop they migrate out to the membranes and seed the organs that create mucus, saliva, tears, and other fluids that protect the membranes. In people whose illnesses let them produce no saliva and so none of the antibodies, tooth decay is quick and ruinous." As a result of this research, several laboratories are attempting to release a vaccine to eliminate tooth decay. This vaccine will stimulate natural antibodies that are present in the saliva. These antibodies destroy the bacteria that cause tooth decay (*Streptococcus mutans*).

Diet

Of course, diet, as is well known, also seriously affects the generation of caries. For example, it has long been known that dental caries occurs in greater numbers of people in regions of the country where rainfall is higher than the average, on the theory that the rainfall washes minerals out of the soil and reduces the amount of minerals found in the local water supply as well as in plants grown on these soils. A deficiency of vitamin A can retard the formation of the matrix of enamel, while vitamin-C deficiency may affect how the collagen matrix is formed. A vitamin-D deficiency often affects the calcification of enamel, dentin, cementum, and alveolar bone. As is well known, dietary carbohydrates in combination with microbial enzymes found on the teeth often promote the development of caries; but of particular interest is the fact that certain microorganisms that require sucrose to survive are among the most important causes of tooth decay in human beings. The best protection against this common disorder is simple: avoid all simple sugars, brush the teeth after every meal, and be certain that a good multivitamin/mineral supplement is provided in your child's diet. Remember this: trace elements may be critical in protecting the bones and teeth. For example, zinc, copper, and molybdenum are essential components of enzymes such as polyphenoloxidase and xanthinoxidase, which are essential to proper tooth function. Conversely, toxic metals such as mercury, lead, and silver inhibit these enzymes. Iron is needed for normal tooth pigmentation, while copper will improve the hardness of enamel. Zinc aids in calcification of the tooth because it activates the alkaline-phosphatase enzyme system, which in turn regulates the laying down of calcium. Molybdenum, which is found in very few vitamin/mineral supplements, especially for children, will protect against caries. This was found in studies that compared children who were raised in areas where the soil was rich in molybdenum with children raised in areas that were poor in molybdenum. It was found that those in areas where the soil is high in molybdenum have less dental caries.

Other interesting mineral relationships include the fact that foods rich in oxalic acid, such as rhubarb, cocoa, and spinach, may interfere with the absorption of calcium by forming insoluble compounds. Similarly, sodium can interfere with the utilization of calcium, while a high intestinal pH can also reduce the absorption of calcium. Of course, bacteria, amino acids, hormones, and vitamins also play major roles in the health or disease of teeth. The purpose of this entry, though, is to show how you can manipulate your child's dietary habits and thereby reduce the risk of tooth decay.

Herbal Preparations:

A cleansing gargle may be prepared from *wild sage,* using ½ teaspoon of the leaves to 1 cup of freshly boiled water. Cover and steep for 5–10 minutes. Allow to cool and use as a gargle and mouthwash.

VOMITING
See REGURGITATION, NAUSEA AND VOMITING

WHOOPING COUGH

Although children are routinely inoculated against whooping cough, this remains a troublesome and potentially dangerous disease for infants and young children. The early stage may be mistaken for a common cold, and so if there is a chance your child has been exposed to whooping cough, *your pediatrician will be needed to help make an early diagnosis.*

The next stage of the disease is marked by a series of rapid consecutive coughs, followed by a deep inhalation with the characteristic whooping sound. There is often vomiting as well, and thick, tenacious mucus that is swallowed or expelled. This stage may last for several weeks, sometimes even months. *Your doctor will need to follow the case closely,* but you can help by providing a nourishing diet, fed in such a way as to encourage retention.

Diet

During the early stage, make every effort to maintain a high-calorie diet, with added, small feedings between meals. If the case is mild, your child will not need to stay in bed, and in fact will do better in fresh air, preferably out of doors; this may also help to maintain appetite.

During the later stage, after the characteristic cough has developed, small, concentrated feedings at frequent intervals are best. Soft, concentrated foods such as cereals, natural puddings, custard, and plain junkets flavored with fruit juice will help avoid irritating the stomach, which may incite coughing. Observe when the coughing spells occur, and arrange to feed your child after a paroxysm of coughing. If vomiting is present, it is easier for your child to keep food down immediately after vomiting.

Infants should be fed in the same way, using thick feedings (see directions on page 150) and solid foods rather than milk mixtures. It is important to maintain fluid intake in all children and infants to prevent dehydration.

Herbal Preparations

To stimulate appetite during the *early stage* of the illness, prepare a tea from one of the following:

Holy Thistle	Place ½ teaspoon of herb in a pot. Add 1 cup freshly boiled water. Cover and steep for 5–10 minutes. Drink warm.
or *Yellow Gentian Root* or *Sweet Fern Root*	Add ½ teaspoon of selected herb to 1½ pints of boiling water. Cover and continue boiling at a slow boil for about 30 minutes. Allow to cool slowly in the closed container. Drink cold, one swallow or 1 tablespoon at a time.

For relief of *cough* during the *later stage,* prepare a tea from one of the following herbs:

Pleurisy Root	Add ½ teaspoon to 1½ pints boiling water. Cover and continue boiling at a slow boil for about 30 minutes. Allow to cool slowly in the closed container. Drink cold, one swallow or 1 tablespoon at a time.
or *Thyme* or *Licorice* or *Maidenhair Fern*	Place ½ teaspoon of selected herb in a pot. Add 1 cup freshly boiled water. Cover and steep for 5–10 minutes. Drink warm.

For relief of *vomiting, red raspberry* is an excellent remedy. Use ½ teaspoon of the *leaf* to a cup of freshly boiled water. Cover and steep for 5–10 minutes. Drink warm. If you use the *root bark*, add ½ teaspoon to 1½ pints of boiling water. Cover and continue boiling at a slow boil for about 30 minutes. Allow to cool slowly in the closed container. Drink cold, one swallow or 1 tablespoon at a time.

BOOK IV
Recipes
for
Resisters

AMERICAN CHILDREN OVERFED YET UNDERNOURISHED

The typical American child suffers from an unexpected ailment that continues to perplex parents, physicians, and dieticians who offer all kinds of rich foods, in great abundance. Our children eat *more* than any other children on earth yet suffer from vitamin and mineral deficiencies, as manifest in a host of physical and emotional complaints, ranging from suicidal thoughts through the gamut of degenerative diseases, including cancer, heart disease, diabetes, mental illness, alcoholism, and so on! Why? The answer, this mysterious disease affecting millions of "well-fed" children, is *malnutrition!*

You see, *over*fed does not equal *well* fed. Fats and sucrose are nutrient-deficient. The nutrient density of these categories of foodstuffs is limited to calories only. They do not contain *any* vitamins or minerals, nor any amino acids, enzymes, or fiber, so desperately needed by growing children, not to speak of overstressed children who are being urged on in their careers from the time they leave the cradle!

TOO MUCH MEAT CAN BE HARMFUL

The majority of our children do eat milk and dairy products, meat, fish, and poultry. These are all good foods provided they come from animals fed naturally and not drugged with hormones and antibiotics that end up in the digestive tracts of the consumer. Of course, all things should be eaten in moderation. And we know that most Americans, including the children, eat far too much meat at the expense of whole grains, fresh fruits, and vegetables. Remember this also: meat is a rich source of phosphorus. Growing children are especially in need of calcium. By overconsuming phosphorus-rich meat we throw the calcium/phosphorus balance out of kilter, setting up long-term metabolic deficits that become increasingly difficult to correct through time.

WHOLESOME RECIPES CAN RESTORE BALANCE

But, returning to the overall picture, we would all do well to reduce our consumption of fats (animal *and* vegetable!), sugar, and dairy products. Note please that we say *reduce,* not eliminate! We need *not* eliminate these foods unless there is a particular allergy or other special dietary reason. To reduce these nutrient categories while increasing our intake of vitamins, minerals, and fiber, all we need do is incorporate some of the recipes that follow. All of these are designed to be made without sugar, fats, oils, eggs, meat, or dairy products. By *supplementing* your family's diet with these recipes, you will increase the nutrient density of your meals while reducing the overconsumed dietary components that are implicated in so many disorders.

CALCIUM SUPPLY MUST BE ASSURED

We must again caution you to be sure that adequate amounts of calcium are supplied in your child's diet, either in the form of supplements (calcium/magnesium tablets or dolomite) or by including calcium-rich foods as outlined on page 83.

WEIMAR KITCHEN YIELDS TASTY, TESTED RECIPES

The following recipes have been created and tested on thousands of satisfied eaters at the Weimar Institute, a healing medical environment in Weimar, California. These are not grim, self-denying recipes but tasty, healthful delights made from simple, wholesome foods. As the cookbook *From the Weimar Kitchen,* the source of these recipes, says:

> Desserts are not forbidden . . . only restricted! From now on . . . God gives you only first-rate gifts wrapped in beautiful natural packages. . . . Eat fewer kinds of food at one meal, and eat with THANKSGIVING.

To this we say, only, Amen.

MISCELLANEOUS

Ingredient Exchange

TO REPLACE	USE
1 c. white flour in baking	1 c. minus 2 t.* whole-wheat flour
1 c. sugar in baking	Omit and try ground-up dates or raisins
1 c. butter, shortening, margarine, or oil in baking	Omit, adding applesauce or water plus 2 T. per c. soy flour in its place

*Capital *T* means *tablespoon(s)* throughout; lower case *t, teaspoon(s)*.

1 egg in baking to bind	1 T. soy or garbanzo flour 3 T. potato flour or tapioca
1 egg in baking to leaven	1 t. baking yeast dissolved in ¼ c. warm water and add 1 T. soy flour to recipe
1 t. baking powder	1–2 t. baking yeast dissolved in ¼ c. warm water

Sautéing Vegetables Without Fat (or Oil)

PLACE a little water in bottom of skillet.
ADD chopped vegetables and cook on low or medium heat until tender. Stir as needed. A little extra water may be added if vegetables become too dry during cooking process.

Preparation of Pans for Baked Goods

PUT a little liquid lecithin on tips of fingers and dab sparsely over surface with fingertips. Then spread with fingers over entire surface of pan as evenly as possible.
WIPE off with a paper towel until there is no trace on a paper towel when wiped over pan.
DUST with finely ground cornmeal.

Preparation of Raw Cashews

Raw cashews are very dirty. They should be washed in lukewarm water and rinsed several times. If they are to be used in a cooked food, it is not necessary to toast them. If they are not to be cooked, as in milk, etc., they should be washed and spread out onto a cookie sheet and put in the oven at 200° or less for 2–3 hrs.

Soy Milk

8 c. water   1 T. vanilla
¾ c. dry soybeans   1 t. salt

BRING water to boil.
BLEND 1 c. of water with ¾ c. dry soybeans. As mixture thickens, add more of the water until blender is full.
POUR blended soybeans in with remainder of water.
POUR through fine strainer.
SIMMER milk for 1 hr. and add vanilla and salt.
COOL and then refrigerate. (Use the bulk in casseroles.)

Chickenlike Seasoning

⅓ c. flour   ½ t. celery salt
¾ t. dry bell-pepper   ½ t. thyme
  powder   ½ t. garlic powder
1 t. onion powder   ¼ t. marjoram
¾ t. salt   1 T. parsley flakes
½ t. sage

DEXTRINIZE ⅓ c. of flour—cornmeal, millet, or barley, etc.—for base (see p. 281).
CHOP ½ bell pepper in fine pieces. Dry in low-heat oven; keep stirring.
GRIND.
MIX all ingredients.

Sprouting Seeds, Beans, and Grain

You can sprout almost any whole natural seed: alfalfa, lentils, mung beans, soybeans, garbanzos, peas, sunflower seeds, wheat, rye, corn, oats, etc. Be sure to buy untreated seeds and grains. These can be obtained in health-food stores. Radish seeds, sprouted, add a zesty flavor to salads.

PUT seeds or grain in glass jar and cover with water.

SOAK overnight. Next morning pour out the water.

RINSE 2–3 times daily until ready to eat, keeping jar covered with a cloth or towel so seeds won't dry out.

Soy and other large beans and lentils, and grains, are best used when the sprouts are short—about ¼″ long. Alfalfa and radish seeds can have longer sprouts. 1 T. alfalfa seed will fill a qt. jar full of sprouts. Use 2 T. seeds when using radish seeds. Use ¼ c. of mung beans. Use ½ c. sunflower, wheat, or rye, etc. Use 1 c. soy or other beans.

BREADS

Basic Whole-Wheat Bread

PUT 2 T. dry yeast in ½ c. warm water. Set the mixture aside to work.

COMBINE 5 c. hot tap water and 7 c. freshly ground whole-wheat flour and 2 T. salt in bowl.

BLEND ¼ c. dates in ½ c. water and add to bowl. Mix until well blended.

ADD 1 c. flour to mixture. Add prepared yeast to mixture and blend thoroughly. Add 4 or 5 more c. flour to mixture. Knead well. If using electric mixer, knead for 10 min. on low speed.

SHAPE into loaves and place dough in pans that have been sprinkled with cornmeal. Let rise ⅓ in bulk (approx. 35 min.).

BAKE at 350° for 35–40 min. Turn out of pans immediately.

Multigrain Bread

5 c. warm water
¾ c. dates
4 c. whole-wheat flour
2 pkgs. yeast
2 T. cashew meal
1 T. salt

4 c. whole-wheat flour
½ c. barley flour
½ c. oatmeal
½ c. cornmeal
½ c. rye flour
½ c. soy flour

LIQUEFY dates in water and add to 4 c. whole-wheat flour and yeast.
STIR well and set in a warm place for 30 min. until bubbly.
ADD remaining ingredients.
KNEAD mixture, adding more whole-wheat flour as needed. Knead for about 10 min. Set in a warm place to rise until double in bulk. Knead down. Let rise until double in bulk again. Form into loaves.
LET rise until nearly double.
BAKE for 10 min. at 425°, then for 40 min. at 375°.
REMOVE immediately from pans and cool on a rack.

Date-Nut Bread

2 c. warm water
1 sweet apple, chopped
2 T. yeast
2 c. whole-wheat flour
1 t. salt

1 c. chopped dates
¾ c. chopped nuts
3–4 c. whole wheat flour

BLEND water with apple until smooth. Add yeast; let sit for a few minutes. Add 2 c. flour to yeast. Beat vigorously. Rise until very light.

ADD salt, dates, nuts, flour, in that order, beating well after each addition.

KNEAD vigorously on well-floured bread board. Rise until light. Mold into 2 loaves.

BAKE in cornmeal-sprinkled pans at 375° for 15 min., then at 350 ° for 45 min.

REMOVE from pan immediately.

Mediterranean Pocket Bread

½ c. boiling water	¼ c. sesame seeds,
2 pitted dates	toasted and ground
1½ c. warm water	5–6 c. whole wheat
2 T. active dry yeast	flour
1 t. salt	4–6 T. cornmeal

SOFTEN dates in ½ c. boiling water for 5 min., then lique-fy in blender. Place in large mixing bowl with 1½ c. warm water.

SPRINKLE yeast over water and let stand 10 min., until foamy. Stir in salt, ground sesame seeds, and 2 c. flour. Beat well for 3 min. Cover and let rise 15 min.

STIR in 2–3 c. more flour, to make a medium-stiff dough.

KNEAD on floured surface for several min., until dough is smooth. Form into long roll and divide dough into 16 equal pieces. Shape each piece into a ball.

PLACE circles of dough on cookie sheets or sheets of foil that have been sprinkled with cornmeal. Cover with waxed paper and let rise 30 min.

PREHEAT oven to 500°. Place circles of dough *directly on bottom rack* of oven.

BAKE at 475° for 5 min.; then turn bread over and bake 1–2 min. more until bread is golden brown all over.

COOL on racks and cover with dry towel. Let cool and air-dry at least 12 hrs. before eating. Cut slit at edge or cut circles in half and stuff with filling.

POCKET BREAD is especially good with hot or cold mashed beans. Garnish with any or all of the following: chopped tomato or cucumber, shredded cabbage, lettuce, carrots, alfalfa sprouts, sliced olives, guacamole.

Crusty Cornbread

1½ c. boiling water
½ c. pitted dates
½ c. raw cashews
1½ t. salt
½ c. warm water
1 T. active dry yeast

1 c. whole-wheat flour, ground fine*
2 c. whole-grain cornmeal, ground fine*

PLACE dates in boiling water in small saucepan. Cover and simmer 15 min. Let stand until lukewarm; then place in blender with cashews and salt.

COVER and whiz at medium speed until smooth. Place ½ c. warm water in large mixing bowl and sprinkle yeast over water. Let stand 10 min., or until foamy.

STIR in date mixture; then stir in flour. With electric mixer (hand mixer works well) beat at medium speed for 5 min.

STIR in cornmeal and beat well. Batter will be stiff.

SPREAD evenly in 8" square *metal* pan that has been sprinkled with cornmeal.†

COVER loosely with foil and let rise in warm place for 40 min.

BAKE at 400° for 1 hr. Cover loosely with foil after first 15 min. of baking to prevent overbrowning top crust. Loosen bread from pan with wide metal spatula; then cool and air-dry on rack at least 12 hrs. before cutting. Reheat in moderate oven before serving.

---

*The finer the flour and cornmeal is ground, the lighter the bread will be.
†Bread can be baked longer in metal pan than in glass baking dish without overbrowning, thus allowing bread to be baked more thoroughly.

BREAKFAST

How to Cook Cereals

Whole-Grain Cookery (wheat and rye)
Bring to rolling boil 1 c. of whole grains and 2½ c. water. Cover and simmer for 1 hr., turn off heat, and let sit overnight. In the morning, simmer until grains burst (about 30–40 min.). Add ½ t. salt when almost done.

Cracked-Grain Cookery (cornmeal, cracked wheat, etc.)
To 1 c. of cereal add about 4 c. cold water and ½–1 t. salt. Place saucepan over fire and stir cereal until it comes to a boil. Cover tightly; reduce heat. In about 20 min. it will be ready to serve with fruit or nuts.

Ground-Grain Cookery
The whole grains should be ground fresh on the day of the breakfast meal preparation. Grind whole grain in Moulinex grinder or blender. The suggested combination is wheat, oats, and rye. Equal amounts of each can be used, or, if preferred, more wheat and oats can be used in proportion to rye. After grinding and mixing the grains, use 1 c. of ground grain to 2½ c. water and ½ t. of salt.

Save out an amount of cold water equal to the amount of grain to mix with the ground grain. Put the rest of the water and the salt in a pan and bring it to a boil. Briskly stir in moistened grain and bring it back to a boil. Turn off heat, cover, and let set about 10–20 min., depending on the amount being prepared. Begin cooking this cereal about 45 min. before serving time.

Pressure-Cooked Wheat
Wash wheat; put in pressure pan; cover with double amount of water. Cook 20 min. at 10 lbs. pressure. Drain and store cooked wheat in freezer for future use.

Crock-Pot Method

1⅓ c. wheat, rye, barley,   2⅔ c. water
   oats, or a combination   1 t. salt

In the evening, place grain, salt, and warm water in crock pot. Turn to low and let it cook all night.

Dextrinized Grains or Flour

Uncooked whole grains such as rice, wheat kernels, rye, oats, cornmeal, cracked wheat, etc., are dextrinized by heating the grain in a heavy skillet until very light brown, stirring constantly to prevent burning. This procedure shortens the cooking time and improves the flavor. (The whole-grain kernels will not necessarily turn brown but will make a popping noise.) Use browned or dextrinized flour for gravies to add flavor and color.

Cashew French Toast

1 c. water   1 T. whole-wheat flour
¾ c. raw cashews   ½ c. fresh orange juice
4 dates   ½ banana
½ t. salt

WHIZ in blender until smooth.
POUR into shallow bowl.
DIP slices of bread into it and place on cookie sheet and
   bake until golden brown.
TURN and brown other side.
TOP with applesauce or fresh fruit.

Mixed-Grain Waffles

4 c. quick oats   1½ t. salt
2 c. whole wheat flour   1 c. water
½ c. soy flour   ⅛ c. cashews
½ c. cornmeal

COMBINE flours and salt.
WHIZ cashews in 1 c. water and then add 6 c. water.
MIX all ingredients well; let stand overnight.
BAKE in hot iron until well browned.
SERVE with fruit sauce.

Granola

1 c. soy flour	½ c. cashews
8 c. rolled oats	1 t. salt
1 c. unsweetened	1½ c. water
shredded coconut	½ c. pitted dates
½ c. sesame seeds, ground	½ c. cashews
1 c. sunflower seeds	1 T. vanilla

COMBINE first 7 ingredients and mix well.
BLEND dates, cashews, and vanilla in water.
POUR into dry mixture and mix well. Spread out on cookie sheets.
BAKE at 200° for 2–3 hrs. or until lightly browned. Stir occasionally for even baking. Raisins (opt.) should be added after baking.

Granola Pudding

MIX 3 c. granola with 3 c. applesauce and let sit overnight in covered baking dish in refrigerator. Before breakfast, add nuts (chopped), and
HEAT 20 min. at 350°.

Almond-Crunch Granola

1 c. boiling water	1 c. fine or medium
1 c. pitted dates, packed	coconut
3 medium or 4 small	½ c. cornmeal or millet
apples	meal

1 t. salt   1 c. wheat flakes*
1 t. vanilla   8 c. rolled oats*
1 c. ground almonds

SCRUB, quarter, and barely remove core from apples.
PLACE dates and apples in boiling water in small sauce-
    pan. Cover and simmer until apples are tender.
GRIND almonds fine in blender and combine with coco-
    nut in large mixing bowl.
WHIZ date mixture with salt and vanilla in blender until
    smooth.
COMBINE with almonds and coconut and beat well.
COOL. When cool, stir in remaining ingredients. CRUM-
    BLE mixture evenly over 2 large cookie sheets, up to 1"
    of edges.
PREHEAT oven to 350°. Place cookie sheets on racks and
REDUCE heat to 250°. Bake for 1 hr., reversing cookie
    sheets on racks after 30 min. to brown granola evenly.
    Stir gently, reduce heat to 200°, and bake 2 hrs. more,
    stirring every 30 min. Reduce oven to lowest heat and
    continue baking until granola is dry and crisp.
COOL and store in airtight container.
    It is easy to overbrown or burn granola, especially at
    the edges. This method of baking should toast granola
    evenly to a golden brown.

MAIN DISHES

How to Cook Dry Beans

MEASURE desired amount of beans (1 c. dry beans yields
    about 2½ c. cooked beans). Remove all particles of
    dirt, sand, or damaged beans. Wash several times, rub-
    bing between palms. You may use a colander for this.

---

*Rolled wheat can replace wheat flakes. 1 c. rolled barley or rolled rye can re-
place 1 c. rolled oats. If desired, grind a few seconds in blender, 1 c. at a time,
to make finer flakes.

COVER with water and soak overnight if desired. Soybeans and garbanzos cook faster if frozen after being soaked. Other beans need not be frozen after being soaked, and may be cooked even without previous soaking. ADD 4 c. water to 1 c. of beans. Use 3 c. water to 1 c. lentils. Bring to boiling point and reduce heat just to keep a constant simmer. Add more boiling water as necessary until beans are at desired tenderness. Lentils may be cooked in less than 1 hr., and should not be soaked; however, other beans may vary up to 2 hrs. or more. (Soybeans and garbanzos will take 5 or more hrs. to be palatable and tender.) When tender, add salt to taste, more or less 1 t. to each c. of dried beans. Additional seasoning is advised as your taste indicates.

Seasoning Suggestions: To all white beans, at the time of salting add a few sprinkles of garlic salt. Lentils and black beans are good this way, too. Simmer for 15 min. more. Red beans and soybeans are tasty with a sauce made of ½ onion diced and sautéed in water. Add 1 clove garlic diced, 1 T. pimento diced, 2 T. tomato sauce (p. 292). (For soybeans use ½ c. tomato sauce and more onion and a bit of fresh lemon juice.) Simmer these together and add to beans. Cook beans until soupy thickness. Pinch of sweet basil may be added for variation. Garbanzos are excellent simmered with chopped onions and a little chicken-like seasoning (p. 275).

Vegetarian Chili Beans

2 c. kidney beans	2½ c. tomatoes
3 c. water	2 t. salt
1 c. chopped onion	1 t. celery seed
1 c. chopped celery	1 garlic clove
½ c. water	

SOAK beans for 24 hrs.
BAKE 3½ hrs. at 250°.
COOK onion and celery in ½ c. water.
ADD to beans.
ADD remaining ingredients and
SIMMER together ½ hr.
SERVE in a ring of cooked brown rice.

Black Beans on Rice

1 lb. black beans	1 bay leaf
1 large onion, chopped	2 t. salt
2 green peppers, chopped	1 lb. brown rice, cooked
½ minced clove garlic	Green onion, chopped

COVER beans with 6 c. boiling water and cook 1 hr.
BRAISE onions, green pepper, and garlic in water.
COMBINE with beans, add other seasonings, and cook un-
   til beans are tender and liquid is thick.
SERVE over brown rice, and sprinkle green onions on top
   of beans

Vegeburgers

4 c. soybeans	Season salt
2 c. garbanzos	Sage
3 c. rice (cooked)	Chickenlike seasoning
6–8 stalks celery	(p. 275)
1–2 onions	Garlic powder
Salt	

SOAK beans overnight; cook, and grind in Moulinex or
   blender.
ADD cooked rice. Sauté celery and onions in a little water.
ADD seasonings.

MIX all together; form patties. If too dry, add bean stock; if too wet, add bread crumbs or oatmeal.

BAKE on Teflon pan at 350°, covered with foil, for about 25 min. If browned, turn, bake about 10 min. more or until browned.

Lentil-Rice Stew

5 c. water
1 c. lentils
½ c. brown rice
1 c. chopped celery tops
1 med. onion, chopped
2 c. potatoes, cubed

2 c. carrots, sliced
1 garlic clove
¼ c. parsley, chopped
    or 1 T. dried parsley
2 t. salt

SIMMER lentils and brown rice until nearly done.
ADD remaining ingredients.
COOK until vegetables are tender.

Almond Loaf

2 c. finely ground
    blanched almonds
2 c. water
1 bunch green onions,
    chopped
½ c. chopped celery
2 t. chickenlike seasoning
    (p. 275)

¼ t. thyme
1 t. leaf basil
½ c. chopped fresh
    parsley
2 c. bread crumbs
Salt to taste

SAUTÉ onions and celery in water until tender.
GRIND almonds finely or liquefy with water in blender until very fine.
COMBINE all ingredients.
BAKE in casserole dish for 1 hr. at 350°. Serve with gravy (see recipes).

Sunflower-Seed Casserole

2 c. sunflower seeds
⅔ c. cashews
¾ c. water
5 c. cooked brown rice

2½ t. chickenlike
    seasoning (p. 275)
1 large *or* 2 small
    onions, chopped fine
⅛ t. garlic powder

GRIND sunflower seeds until fine.
BLEND cashews and water until smooth.
COMBINE all ingredients and mix thoroughly. Put into
    large casserole and
BAKE for 1½ hrs., at 325°.
LEAVE cover on casserole for first 45 min.

Eggplant Casserole Deluxe

SLICE eggplant very thin. Roll slices in a breading mix-
    ture of cornmeal and garlic salt.
PLACE breaded slices on cookie sheet in very hot oven
    (450–500°) for about 15–25 min.
CUT onions and bell peppers into rings.
MAKE a sauce with tomato sauce (p. 292) and pimiento.
ARRANGE eggplant slices in bottom of casserole dish,
    then
ADD a layer of onions and bell pepper slices, and sauce,
    and repeat until dish is full.
BAKE in oven at 400° until done.

Crunchy Nut Lentil Roast

2 c. cooked lentils
1½ c. onion, sautéed in
    water
1½ c. cooked brown rice
½ c. chopped celery

½ c. chopped walnuts
    (opt.)
1 t. rubbed sage
1 t. salt
½ t. marjoram

MIX cooked lentils and rice.
ADD all other ingredients.
PUT in baking dish and
BAKE at 350° for 30–45 min.

Garbanzo-Rice Patties

1½ c. garbanzos, cooked
1½ c. cooked brown rice
¾ c. water

½ onion, chopped fine
1 t. salt
⅛ t. garlic powder

BLEND garbanzos with water until smooth. Add remaining ingredients, except rice, and blend well.
POUR into bowl and add rice, mixing well. Drop by teaspoonfuls onto cookie sheet and
BAKE for 30 min. at 325°. May be baked in casserole for 30 min. covered and for another 30 min. uncovered at 325°.

Saucy-Soy Sizzlers in Tomato Sauce

½ c. dry soybeans
1 c. water
1 c. rolled oats
1 c. celery

½ c. chopped nuts
1 med. onion
½ t. salt

SOAK soybeans overnight in 3 c. water.
DRAIN and whiz in blender with 1 c. water until fine. Pour into bowl.
ADD rolled oats and let stand 10 min.
ADD remaining ingredients. Mix well.
FORM into patties and place on cookie sheet that has been sprinkled with cornmeal.
BROWN lightly in oven.
MAKE a tomato sauce (p. 292) and pour over the sizzlers.
BAKE in 350° oven 20–30 min.

Cabbage Rolls

1 med. head cabbage	½ t. celery salt
½ c. chopped celery	¼ t. sage
½ c. chopped onion	¼ t. garlic salt
¼ c. chopped green	1 c. cooked brown rice
pepper	¼ c. water
1 c. tomato sauce (p. 292)	

STEAM cabbage until leaves can be removed easily.
SIMMER vegetables in water until nearly tender.
ADD seasoning. Simmer a few minutes more and add to cooked rice.
MIX well. Put ½ cup rice mixture in cabbage leaf and roll.
PLACE in baking pan and pour tomato sauce and water over them.
BAKE 45 min. at 350°.

NOTE: Can add extra tomato sauce to rice mixture before putting into cabbage leaves to make more moist. Can use this mixture for stuffed zucchini or peppers as well.

Stuffed Green Peppers

1 c. canned tomatoes	½ t. sweet basil
½ c. tomato sauce (p. 292)	2 t. sage
3 stalks celery, chopped	¼ t. garlic powder
3 onions, chopped	1 t. thyme
1½ t. salt	6 c. cooked brown rice

SIMMER together tomatoes, celery, and onion until fairly dry and barely tender.
ADD remaining ingredients.
MIX all ingredients and add enough bread crumbs to make dry mixture. Unless the peppers are parboiled they make the mixture quite moist while baking.

PACK loosely into raw, stemmed, and cored peppers.
BAKE at 400° for 50 min. covered, 10 min. uncovered. (1
T. of water should be put in bottom of baking dish to
give moisture until peppers form their own.)

Cashew-Tomato Chow Mein

3 med. onions, sliced in rings	3–4 med. tomatoes, cut in wedges
3–4 stalks celery, cut on slant	½ c. lightly toasted cashews
2 c. Chinese pea pods (sugar peas)	Onion and garlic salt, to taste
2 c. mung bean sprouts	

PLACE just enough water in large skillet with tight-fitting
lid to cook vegetables without going dry (¼–½ c.).
SPRINKLE in onion and garlic salt to taste; then bring water to boil.
PLACE onion rings in skillet and place celery and pea
pods evenly over onions.
COVER and cook over high heat until steam escapes.
REDUCE heat to simmer and cook 5 min., or until celery
and pea pods are tender.
TOSS in bean sprouts, cashews, and tomato wedges and
serve at once.
SERVE over steaming brown rice. Long-grain brown rice
is especially good with vegetables.

YIELD: 4 generous servings.

Corn-Tamale Bake

1 large onion, chopped	¼ c. chopped olives
1 green pepper, chopped	3 cloves garlic
3 c. canned tomatoes	¾ c. cornmeal
2 c. corn, drained	Salt to taste

SAUTÉ onion and pepper in water.
ADD all other ingredients.
SIMMER in covered skillet for 1 hr.
STIR occasionally and add a little water if it gets too thick
  (up to ¾ c. water).
PUT in baking dish to warm over.

GRAVIES AND SAUCES

Brown Gravy

2 c. water (potato or green
  bean if available)
4 Brazil nuts
¼ t. fine herbs
⅛ t. garlic

½ c. whole wheat flour,
  dextrinized (see p.
  281)
¾ t. salt

WHIZ all ingredients in blender.
BRING to boil on medium heat, stirring constantly.
SIMMER 10 min.

Golden Sauce

¾ c. cooked potato
1 med. carrot, cooked
1⅓ c. water

2 T. cashews
¾ t. salt
1 T. fresh lemon juice

BLEND in blender until smooth.
HEAT and
SERVE over vegetables such as cauliflower, broccoli, egg-
  plant, etc.

Vegetable Gravy

6 c. water
1 small potato
1 small onion
1 stalk celery

⅛ t. thyme
⅛ t. sage
⅛ t. garlic powder

COOK together until vegetables are done.
MASH vegetables. May add arrowroot to thicken.

Cashew Gravy or White Sauce

2 c. hot water
½ c. cashews

Onion salt to taste

WHIZ in blender until smooth.
POUR into small pan and bring to boil.
USE as gravy for potatoes or as a white sauce.

Tomato Sauce

2 28-oz. cans whole
  tomatoes *or* 2 qts. home-
  canned tomatoes
4 cloves garlic *or* ½ t.
  garlic powder
1 c. carrot, cut up

2 c. celery with leaves,
  cut up
2 c. fresh onion, cut up,
  or 1 c. dried onion
  flakes
½ t. salt (to taste)

DRAIN liquid from tomatoes into blender.
ADD garlic, carrot, and whiz at high speed until liquefied.
ADD celery and chop fine. If using fresh onion, add onion
  and chop. Pour into large saucepan. In blender,
CHOP tomatoes a few seconds at low speed and pour into
  saucepan. If using dried onion flakes, stir in.
BRING to boil, cover, and

SIMMER 1 hr. Add salt to taste. If possible, let stand overnight for flavors to blend. Sauce freezes well.

This sauce is delicious with enchiladas, lasagna, stuffed
peppers, patties, or wherever a flavorful tomato sauce
is needed. Carrots and celery add delicious flavor as
well as valuable nutrients.

For pizza sauce, use dried onion flakes as they thicken
sauce much more than fresh onion. Home-dried tomato slices can also be used to thicken tomato sauce.
Grind dried tomato slices to powder in dry blender. $\frac{1}{2}$
c. powder will thicken sauce nicely. Stir in after sauce
has simmered for 1 hr. Increase seasoning to taste. Let
stand for flavors to blend.

The best-quality tomatoes are used in canned whole tomatoes. Commercially canned tomato products such as
tomato paste, tomato puree, and tomato sauce are not
recommended, because they may have been prepared
from spoiled or moldy tomatoes.

DRESSINGS AND SPREADS

No-Oil Soy Mayonnaise

PLACE 1½ c. water in pan and bring to a boil. Then thor-
oughly mix 3 T. arrowroot powder in 1½ c. water.
ADD this to the boiling water and bring to a boil again.
REMOVE from heat. Place 1 c. of water in blender.
ADD to this 1 c. of soy milk (p. 275) and 2 c. raw cashews
and blend thoroughly.
ADD ¾ c. lemon juice, 1 T. salt, and 2 t. garlic powder
and blend.
ADD starch mixture and mix thoroughly.
RERIGERATE.

Creamy Lemon Dressing

1 c. water
2 T. arrowroot powder
½ c. sunflower seeds
⅛ t. ground dill seed
⅛ t. onion powder

⅛ t. garlic powder
⅛ t. celery seed
½ t. Vegesal *or* ¼ t. salt
¼ c. fresh lemon juice

BLEND together water and arrowroot.
SIMMER until thickened and put in blender (cool first if necessary).
ADD remaining ingredients.
BLEND until smooth.

Coleslaw Dressing

½–1 c. cashews
1 small cucumber
1 small onion
1 t. onion salt

4 t. fresh lemon juice
Water for desired thickness

BLEND and
POUR over salad.

Bean Spread

2 c. cooked beans, drained
6 T. tomato sauce (page 292)

½ t. onion salt
⅛ t. sweet basil
⅛ t. garlic powder

BLEND beans until smooth, adding enough bean liquid to make a thick puree.
POUR puree into top of double boiler.
ADD remaining ingredients.
(GRIND the herbs into a powder before adding.)
COOK until the mixture is thoroughly heated, stirring frequently.
CHILL.

Hommus Tahini

2 c. cooked garbanzos	1 T. chopped parsley
1/2 c. sesame seed	(opt.)
1 clove garlic (opt.)	3 T. fresh lemon juice
Salt to taste	

LIQUEFY beans, salt (about 1/2 t. if garbanzos are unsalted), garlic, and seed, with barely enough bean broth to make blender turn.
SPRINKLE with garlic powder if clove garlic is omitted.
SERVE over toast.

Don's Fruit Butter

1 c. unsweetened crushed pineapple	1/4 c. coconut (unsweetened, finely shredded)
3 peaches, fresh	1/2 c. walnuts
1 banana	3–4 dates

BLEND all ingredients in blender except nuts.
ADD nuts at the end and
WHIZ just enough to leave a little chunky.
Delicious over waffles, cereal or toast. Keep in refrigerator.

VARIATIONS: In place of peaches, use apricots, apples or persimmons.

Nut or Seed Butter

PUT 1/2 c. water in blender.
ADD nuts of any kind to blender until the desired consistency of butter is reached.
ADD a pinch of salt and flavorings if desired.
USE sparingly.

ALTERNATE: grind nuts or seeds in nut grinder until fine. Pour into container and add enough water to make a thick paste.

VARIATION: Almonds, cashews, walnuts, peanuts, hazel nuts, sesame seeds, sunflower seeds, etc. Nuts or seeds could be *lightly* roasted.

Dried-Fruit Jam

REHYDRATE dried apples, pears, peaches, etc., *or* any combination of these with just enough water to cover the fruit.

SIMMER until soft or soak overnight.

PUT in blender and whiz until smooth.

STORE in refrigerator. (Will keep at least a week.)

INCREASE sweetness by adding date granules simmered in small amount of water until soft, or chopped pitted dates.

BLEND all together until smooth.

Jams

Peanut-Pineapple Jam
Dilute peanut butter with water and then add crushed pineapple.

Apple Jam
Soak 1 c. dried apples and ½ c. dates in 3 c. water and then blend.

Fig Jam
Blend dried figs with desired amount of fresh orange juice.

Prune Jam
2 c. pitted prunes, 1 c. cashew nuts. Add water and blend.

Almond-Date Jam
Blend almonds and dates with equal amount of water.

Pineapple-Apricot Jam
1¼ c. pitted dried prunes *or* 1 c. pitted dates, 1 c. dried apricots, and ½ c. crushed unsweetened pineapple. Simmer prunes and apricots in water (enough to cover fruit) until soft, or soak overnight. Blend with pineapple in blender until smooth.

VEGETABLES

Best Methods for Cooking Vegetables

COOK without water, if possible.
COOK as short a time as possible and just before serving.
AVOID bruising, soaking, or wilting vegetables.
KEEP vegetables cold until ready to cook.
AVOID use of soda for preserving color and crispness.
DO NOT remove cover while cooking.
AVOID the use of utensils that are chipped, worn, or have copper alloys.
USE plastic scouring pad or stiff brush for vegetables, not a metal-mesh pad.
WHEN DONE, vegetables should have a crisp, tender texture. Overcooked they are mushy, strong flavored, and lose attractive natural color.
COOK vegetables whole or in large pieces when possible. Cook with skins on to save nutrients.
START vegetables in boiling water to conserve the greatest possible amount of nutrients. To preserve the bright green color, cook vegetables uncovered for 1 min. *After* boiling point has been reached, cover, reduce heat promptly to lowest cooking level, and cook until done.
STIR as little as possible, and do not boil vigorously.
A SMALL amount of fresh lemon juice added to the cooking water will help restore the color of red cabbage and beets.

SERVE as soon as the vegetable is cooked. Keeping vegetables warm after they are cooked causes loss of food value, particularly vitamins. If they must wait, allow to cool, then reheat.

Baked Stuffed Potatoes

5 med. potatoes
1 T. parsley
1 T. chives (opt.)

¾ c. no-oil soy
  mayonnaise (p. 293)
Salt to taste

SCRUB potatoes.
BAKE at 400° for 1 hr. or until tender.
CUT a slice from top of each lengthwise. Scoop out insides, being careful not to break shell. Mash the potatoes in a mixing bowl and add remaining ingredients. Lightly
SPOON this mixture back into the potato shells.
SPRINKLE top with paprika and
BAKE for 15 min. at 400°.

Vegetable Casserole

2 c. grated carrot
2 c. chopped celery
1 c. ground raw sunflower
  seeds
½ c. shredded cabbage *or*
  chopped chard *or*
  spinach
2 t. fresh lemon juice
1 t. minced onion

⅛ t. garlic powder
Salt to taste
1 t. ground bell pepper
  (dry)
1 t. dried parsley
Thick gravy to moisten,
  about 1 c. (see
  recipes)

MIX together with gravy.
PRESS into loaf pan.
BAKE at 350° until vegetables are tender.

Green-Bean Casserole

USE either fresh or frozen green beans.
COOK until tender. (Follow instructions on package if frozen beans are used.) Drain.
ADD ¼ c. chopped cashews or almonds to each 2 c. of beans.
POUR into a casserole and cover with a white sauce (p. 292) to which has been added 1 t. of chickenlike seasoning (p. 275) per c. of sauce.
SPRINKLE with seasoned bread crumbs.
BAKE for 20 min. at 350°.

Zucchini-Corn Scallop

2 lbs. zucchini	1 c. whole kernel corn
3 green onions, minced	1 c. canned tomatoes
¼ c. chopped green pepper	Salt to taste
	2 T. minced parsley

SCRUB zucchini and slice into ¼" pieces. Put into skillet with onion, green pepper, corn, and small amount water. Cook gently.
ADD tomatoes and cook until hot.
ADD salt to taste.
POUR into a 1½ qt. casserole, sprinkle top with parsley.
BAKE in a 350° oven for 30 min. until heated through.
YIELD: 6 servings.

Oriental-Style Broccoli

3 med. onions, sliced in rings	½ c. toasted almonds, whole or slivered
1 bunch fresh broccoli	Onion and garlic salt, to taste
3–4 med. tomatoes, cut in wedges	

PREPARE broccoli by rinsing well in cold running water.

CUT away tough stalks and slice remaining stalks ¼″ thick up to where broccoli head divides into small sections.

CUT sections into size suitable for serving.

PLACE in large skillet with tight-fitting lid with just enough water to cook vegetables without going dry (¼–½ c.).

SPRINKLE in onion and garlic salt to taste; then bring to boil. Place onion rings in skillet and place broccoli evenly over onion rings.

COVER and cook over high heat until steam escapes.

REDUCE heat to simmer and cook 5 min. or until broccoli is tender.

TOSS in almonds and tomato wedges and serve at once. If broccoli is covered after it is cooked, it will turn brownish green in color.

YIELD: 4 servings.

Rosy Crunch Salad

1 c. shredded carrots   Green-pepper strips
1 c. shredded beets   Endive
1 c. shredded turnips

MAKE a mound of each vegetable.

PRESS together into 1 mound.

DECORATE top with alfalfa sprouts and strips of green pepper.

DECORATE base with endive.

VARIATION: The vegetables may be tossed with dressing.

Carrot Salad

2 carrots, shredded fine   ¼ c. walnuts, chopped,
½ c. celery, chopped   or ¼ c. coconut, med.
                                         unsweetened

MIX and
SERVE.

Potato Salad

6 med. cold precooked
  potatoes with peelings
1 c. celery, diced
1 c. olives, chopped
½ c. pimiento, chopped
2–3 t. onion powder
1 T. dried parsley flakes

1 T. ground dill seed *or*
  dill weed
Salt to taste
  (approx. 2 t.)
Paprika for color
1 c. no-oil soy
  mayonnaise (p. 293)

MIX potatoes with celery.
ADD pimiento and olives.
ADD seasonings and
MIX thoroughly. Then
ADD no-oil soy mayonnaise and mix thoroughly.
LET set overnight for better flavor.

SOUPS

Garden-Vegetable Soup

2 med. potatoes, diced
2 med. carrots, diced
1 c. string beans, cut small
1 med. onion, diced
2 med. summer squash,
  diced
2 large stalks celery, diced
3 med. tomatoes, cut in
  small pieces

¼ large green pepper,
  diced
2 t. salt
1 t. onion salt
1 T. parsley
¼ t. thyme
¼ t. sweet basil
¼ t. marjoram
⅛ t. dill weed
⅛ t. garlic salt

PUT vegetables into a large saucepan and cover with approx. 2½ qts. water.
BRING to a boil and add seasoning to taste. Continue to simmer until vegetables are nearly cooked.
ADD either pearl barley, brown rice, or whole-wheat spaghetti and continue to cook until done.

Minestrone

1 c. garbanzo beans
2 small onions, chopped
    fine
2 stalks celery, chopped
    fine
1 small can tomatoes,
    mashed
2 zucchini, sliced thin
1 carrot, shredded

2 garlic cloves, chopped
1 bay leaf
1 pinch thyme, minced
1 pinch savory, minced
⅛ t. marjoram, minced
⅛ t. rosemary, minced
½ green pepper,
    chopped fine
⅛ t. basil, minced

SOAK beans overnight in 1 qt. water.
COOK beans 20 min. at 15 lbs. in pressure cooker (or for
    50 min.).
COOK remaining ingredients in 1 pint water until done.
COMBINE all ingredients.
ADD 1½ qts. water and heat to boiling.

Lentil Soup

1 lg. or 2 med. chopped
    onions
4 cloves minced garlic
3 c. lentils (1 lb.)
2 qts. water

1 qt. tomatoes
1 t. salt
½ t. dill seed
2 bay leaves

COOK lentils, onions, and garlic in water for 40 min.
ADD tomatoes, salt, and seasonings.
COOK 20–40 min. more.

This soup tastes even better when made ahead!

SWEET THINGS

Apple-Pie Filling

8 apples
2 T. arrowroot powder
½ c. raisins
½ c. dates, chopped

½ T. coriander
½ t. anise
Pinch of salt

PEEL and core apples.
COOK with raisins and dates until tender.
ADD other ingredients.
STIR and cook until clear.
POUR into baked pie shell.

No-Oil Pie Crust

1 c. cashews
½ t. salt

½ c. water
1 c. whole-wheat flour

BLEND cashews, water, and salt until smooth.
ADD flour to make soft pastry dough.
PRESS into pie pan and
BAKE at 375° until done.

Apple-Prune Betty

2 c. sliced apples
1 c. stewed prunes
⅓ c. fresh lemon juice
¼ t. coriander

1½ c. bread crumbs
½ c. liquid from stewed
   prunes.

ARRANGE apples, prunes, and crumbs in layers in baking
   dish. Just before adding the top layer of crumbs, pour
   the prune liquid and lemon juice combined over all.
BAKE at 350° until apples are tender, and serve hot.

Tropical Rice

4 c. water
1 c. brown rice
1 c. soy or nut cream
  (blend ½ c. water and
  ½ c. nuts)
¼ c. coconut,
  unsweetened

¾ c. dates, chopped
1 14-oz. can pineapple
  pieces, unsweetened
2 bananas, sliced

BRING water and rice to boil.
SIMMER 1 hr. or until all liquid is absorbed.
STIR occasionally.
ADD cream.
MIX, cover, and cool until warm.
ADD remaining ingredients.
MIX lightly.
SERVE immediately.
YIELD: serves 6–8.

"Chocolate" Ice Cream

5 dates
¾ c. water
¼ t. salt
½ c. cashews

2 T. carob powder
1½ t. vanilla
4–5 frozen ripe bananas

BLEND together and slowly add bananas. Don't overload
  the blender.
POUR into container and freeze or eat immediately as
  soft ice cream.

Fruit Leather

BLEND any very ripe fruit with a very small amount of
  water. A ripe banana may be added if fruits are very
  tart.
LINE a flat pan with plastic wrap.

POUR fruit on pan and spread to ¼" thickness or thinner.
PLACE in warm oven at 125°, with oven door slightly
    ajar. If sun is hot, may place in sun for 2 or 3 days.
    When you can pick it up and remove it from plastic
    easily, it is dry enough (approx. 12 hrs.).
CUT in squares or roll if desired. Children enjoy tearing
    off a piece for a wholesome dessert.

Banana-Date Cookies

1 c. boiling water
1 c. pitted dates
¾ t. salt
1 t. vanilla
1 t. fresh lemon juice

1 c. chopped walnuts
4 med. or 3 large very
    ripe bananas, barely
    mashed (about 2 c.)
4 c. rolled oats*

CHOP walnuts in blender just a few seconds, then place in
    a large mixing bowl.
PLACE dates in boiling water in small saucepan. Cover
    and
SIMMER 15 min. In blender,
WHIZ date mixture with salt, vanilla, and lemon juice un-
    til smooth. Combine with walnuts,
STIR in mashed bananas. Stir in oats and mix well. Drop
    by teaspoonfuls onto 2 large Teflon cookie sheets and
    flatten with fork.
BAKE at 325° for 30 min.; then reduce heat to 225° and
    bake 30 min. longer. Reverse cookie sheets on oven
    racks every 15 min. during baking to brown cookies
    evenly.
YIELD: About 5 dozen.

Because they contain so much fresh and dried fruit, these
cookies will soften after standing. If desired, before
serving, reheat in moderate oven for "just-baked"
crispness, flavor, and aroma.

*Quaker Old Fashioned rolled oats (5-min.) are best for these cookies. Some
rolled oats have thicker flakes and do not blend as nicely into cookies.

Carob-Fudge Cookies

3 med. *or* 4 small apples
1½ c. pitted dates
1 c. boiling water
1 t. salt
1 t. fresh lemon juice

1 c. lightly toasted
  almonds
¾ c. carob powder,
  sifted
½ c. coconut
3 c. rolled oats

SCRUB, quarter, and barely remove core from apples.

PLACE dates and apples in boiling water in small saucepan.

COVER and simmer until apples are tender. In blender coarsely chop almonds.

SIFT carob powder into large mixing bowl and combine with almonds and coconut. In blender, whiz date mixture until smooth with salt and lemon juice. Place in mixing bowl and beat well.

STIR in oats and mix well.

DROP by teaspoonfuls onto 2 large nonstick cookie sheets.

FLATTEN cookies with fork.

BAKE at 325° for 30 min., reversing cookie sheets on oven racks after 15 min. to brown cookies evenly.

For brownies, spread cookie mixture in 9" × 13" baking dish that has been prepared with liquid lecithin. Bake at 325° for 40 min.

Chilled orange slices with carob cookies or brownies make a delightful dessert!

Rita's Apple Crisp

1½ c. rolled oats
1½ c. whole-wheat flour
½ c. chopped dates
½ t. salt
½ c. cashew cream
  (p. 307)

½ c. chopped nuts
10 apples sliced
1 20-oz. can pineapple
2 T. arrowroot powder
¼ t. ground coriander
¼ t. ground sweet anise

BLEND pineapple and set aside.
COMBINE dry ingredients and
ADD cashew cream and ½ c. blended pineapple.
HEAT apples and dates and
STIR in coriander, anise, and arrowroot blended in remainder of pineapple.
POUR apples in baking dish and drop topping in chunks on top and pat down.
BAKE at 350° until apples bubble and top browns.

Cashew-Nut Cream

¾ c. raw cashews or   6–8 dates
    almonds   ½ t. vanilla
1 c. water   Pinch of salt

BLEND until smooth. Will thicken in refrigerator.

Strawberry Cream

1½ c. water (cold)   ¼ c. dates
½ c. cashews   Pinch of salt
½ c. cooked rice   1 t. fresh lemon juice
1 c. frozen strawberries

BLEND all ingredients.
CHILL until served.

VARIATIONS: Use any other frozen fruit in place of strawberries.

APPENDIX A

1980 Revised Recommended Dietary Allowances

Recommended Dietary Allowances, Revised 1980*
Designed for the maintenance of good nutrition of practically
all healthy people in the U.S.A.
Food and Nutrition Board, National Academy of
Sciences–National Research Council

Age and Sex Group	Weight		Height		Protein	Fat-Soluble Vitamins			Water-Soluble Vitamins		
	kg.	lb.	cm.	in.		Vitamin A	Vitamin D	Vitamin E	Vitamin C	Thiamine	Ribo-flavin
					gm.	$\mu g.R.E.$†	$\mu g.$‡	$mg.\alpha T.E.$#		mg.	
Infants											
0.0-0.5 yr.	6	13	60	24	kg.×2.2	420	10	3	35	0.3	0.4
0.5-1.0 yr.	9	20	71	28	kg.×2.0	400	10	4	35	0.5	0.6
Children											
1-3 yr.	13	29	90	35	23	400	10	5	45	0.7	0.8
4.6 yr.	20	44	112	44	30	500	10	6	45	0.9	1.0
7-10 yr.	28	62	132	52	34	700	10	7	45	1.2	1.4
Males											
11-14 yr.	45	99	157	62	45	1,000	10	8	50	1.4	1.6
15-18 yr.	66	145	176	69	56	1,000	10	10	60	1.4	1.7
19-22 yr.	70	154	177	70	56	1,000	7.5	10	60	1.5	1.7
23-50 yr.	70	154	178	70	56	1,000	5	10	60	1.4	1.6
51+ yr.	70	154	178	70	56	1,000	5	10	60	1.2	1.4
Females											
11-14 yr.	46	101	157	62	46	800	10	8	50	1.1	1.3
15-18 yr.	55	120	163	64	46	800	10	8	60	1.1	1.3
19-22 yr.	55	120	163	64	44	800	7.5	8	60	1.1	1.3
23-50 yr.	55	120	163	64	44	800	5	8	60	1.0	1.2
51+ yr.	55	120	163	64	44	800	5	8	60	1.0	1.2
Pregnancy					+30	+200	+5	+2	+20	+0.4	+0.3
Lactation					+20	+400	+5	+3	+40	+0.5	+0.5

*The allowances are intended to provide for individual variations among most normal persons as they live in the United States under usual environmental stresses. Diets should be based on a variety of common foods in order to provide other nutrients for which human requirements have been less well defined. See text for detailed discussion of allowances and of nutrients not tabulated. See preceding table for weights and heights by individual year of age and for suggested average energy intakes.

†Retinol equivalents; 1 retinol equivalent = 1μg. retinol or 6μg. β-carotene. See text for calculation of vitamin activity of diets as retinol equivalents.

‡As cholescalciferol: 10 μg. cholecalciferol = 400 I.U. vitamin D.

#α tocopherol equivalents: 1 mg. d-α-tocopherol = 1αT.E. See text for variation in allowances and calculation of vitamin E activity of the diet as α tocopherol equivalents.

¶1 N.E. (niacin equivalent) = 1 mg. niacin or 60 mg dietary tryptophan.

[308]

	Water-Soluble Vitamins					Minerals			
Niacin	Vitamin B₆	Folacin§	Vitamin B₁₂	Calcium	Phosphorus	Magnesium	Iron	Zinc	Iodine
mg.N.E.¶	mg.	µg.				mg.			µg.
6	0.3	30	0.5**	360	240	50	10	3	40
8	0.6	45	1.5	540	360	70	15	5	50
9	0.9	100	2.0	800	800	150	15	10	70
11	1.3	200	2.5	800	800	200	10	10	90
16	1.6	300	3.0	800	800	250	10	10	120
18	1.8	400	3.0	1,200	1,200	350	18	15	150
18	2.0	400	3.0	1,200	1,200	400	18	15	150
19	2.2	400	3.0	800	800	350	10	15	150
18	2.2	400	3.0	800	800	350	10	15	150
16	2.2	400	3.0	800	800	350	10	15	150
15	1.8	400	3.0	1,200	1,200	300	18	15	150
14	2.0	400	3.0	1,200	1,200	300	18	15	150
14	2.0	400	3.0	800	800	300	18	15	150
13	2.0	400	3.0	800	800	300	18	15	150
13	2.0	400	3.0	800	800	300	10	15	150
+2	+0.6	+400	+1.0	+400	+400	+150	††	+ 5	+25
+5	+0.5	+100	+1.0	+400	+400	+150	††	+10	+50

§The folacin allowances refer to dietary sources as determined by *Lactobacillus casei* assay after treatment with enzymes ("conjugases") to make polyglutamyl forms of the vitamin available to the test organism.

**The RDA for vitamin B₁₂ in infants is based on average concentration of the vitamin in human milk. The allowances after weaning are based on energy intake (as recommended by the American Academy of Pediatrics) and consideration of other factors, such as intestinal absorption; see text.

††The increased requirement during pregnancy cannot be met by the iron content of habitual American diets or by the existing iron stores of many women; therefore, the use of 30 to 60 mg. supplemental iron is recommended. Iron needs during lactation are not substantially different from those of non-pregnant women, but continued supplementation of the mother for two to three months after parturition is advisable in order to replenish stores depleted by pregnancy.

[309]

Estimated safe and adequate daily dietary intakes of additional selected vitamins and minerals*

Age Group	Vitamins			Trace Elements†		
	Vitamin K	Biotin	Pantothenic Acid	Copper	Manganese	Fluoride
	µg.					
Infants						
0.0-0.5 yr.	12	35	2	0.5-0.7	0.5-0.7	0.1-0.5
0.5-1.0 yr.	10- 20	50	3	0.7-1.0	0.7-1.0	0.2-1.0
Children and adolescents						
1-3 yr.	15- 30	65	3	1.0-1.5	1.0-1.5	0.5-1.5
4-6 yr.	20- 40	85	3-4	1.5-2.0	1.5-2.0	1.0-2.5
7-10 yr.	30- 60	120	4-5	2.0-2.5	2.0-3.0	1.5-2.5
11+ yr.	50-100	100-200	4-7	2.0-3.0	2.5-5.0	1.5-2.5
Adults	70-140	100-200	4-7	2.0-3.0	2.5-5.0	1.5-4.0

*From Recommended Dietary Allowances. Revised 1980. Food and Nutrition Board, National Academy of Sciences—National Research Council. Because there is less information on which to base allowances, these figures are not given in the main table of the RDAs and are provided here in the form of ranges

Trace Elements†			Electrolytes		
Chromium	Selenium	Molybdenum	Sodium	Potassium	Chloride

mg.

0.01-0.04	0.01-0.04	0.03-0.06	115- 350	350- 925	275- 700
0.02-0.06	0.02-0.06	0.04-0.08	250- 750	425-1,275	400-1,200
0.02-0.08	0.02-0.08	0.05-0.1	325- 975	550-1,650	500-1,500
0.03-0.12	0.03-0.12	0.06-0.15	450-1,350	775-2,325	700-2,100
0.05-0.2	0.05-0.2	0.1 -0.3	600-1,800	1,000-3,000	925-2,775
0.05-0.2	0.05-0.2	0.15-0.5	900-2,700	1,525-4,575	1,400-4,200
0.05-0.2	0.05-0.2	0.15-0.5	1,100-3,300	1,875-5,625	1,700-5,100

of recommended intakes.

†Since the toxic levels for many trace elements may be only several times usual intakes, the upper levels for the trace elements given in this table should not be habitually exceeded.

APPENDIX B

Longevity Formula

(An "ideal" broad-spectrum multivitamin/mineral
formula for children)*

	Dosage		
	3 Tabs Age 10–14	2 Tabs Age 5–9	1 Tab Age 2–4
Vitamin A (Fish Liver Oil)	7,500 I.U.	5,000 I.U.	2,500 I.U.
Vitamin D₃ (Cholecalciferol)	100 I.U.	66.6 I.U.	33.3 I.U.
Vitamin E (d-alpha Tocopherol Succinate)	90 I.U.	60 I.U.	30 I.U.
Vitamin C (Mineral Ascorbates)	500 mg.	333.3 mg.	166.6 mg.
Folic Acid	150 mcg.	100 mcg.	50 mcg.
Thiamine (Vitamin B₁)	30 mg.	20 mg.	10 mg.
Riboflavin (Vitamin B₂)	30 mg.	20 mg.	10 mg.
Niacinamide	30 mg.	20 mg.	10 mg.
Vitamin B₆ (Pyridoxine HCl)	30 mg.	20 mg.	10 mg.
Vitamin B₁₂ (Cyanocabalamin)	7.5 mcg.	5 mcg.	2.5 mcg.
Biotin	100 mcg.	66.6 mcg.	33.3 mcg.
Pantothenic Acid	30 mg.	20 mg.	10 mg.
Calcium (Ascorbate)	50 mg.	33.3 mg.	16.6 mg.
Phosphorus (Bonemeal)	25 mg.	16.6 mg.	8.3 mg.
Iodine (Kelp)	15 mcg.	10 mcg.	5 mcg.
Iron (Peptonate)	5 mg.	3.3 mg.	1.6 mg.
Magnesium (Citrate, Ascorbate)	50 mg.	33.3 mg.	16.6 mg.
Copper (Gluconate)	25 mcg.	16.6 mcg.	8.3 mcg.
Zinc (Ascorbate)	7.5 mg.	5 mg.	2.5 mg.
Chromium (Yeast)	15 mcg.	10 mcg.	5 mcg.
Manganese (Ascorbate)	2.5 mg.	1.6 mg.	0.8 mg.
Molybdenum	15 mcg.	10 mcg.	5 mcg.
Potassium (Proteinate)	25 mg.	16.6 mg.	8.3 mg.
Selenium (Yeast)	15 mcg.	10 mcg.	5 mcg.
RNA (Ribonucleic Acid)	30 mg.	20 mg.	10 mg.
Lecithin	100 mg.	66.6 mg.	33.3 mg.
Choline	18 mg.	12 mg.	6 mg.
Inositol	18 mg.	12 mg.	6 mg.
PABA (Para-aminobenzoic Acid)	18 mg.	12 mg.	6 mg.
Citrus Bioflavonoids	150 mg.	100 mg.	50 mg.
Hesperidin	60 mg.	40 mg.	20 mg.

*A commercially available source of this formula is "Omni Junior," available
from DaVinci Laboratories, South Burlington, Vt. 05401.

Selected Bibliography

Bayless, T.M., I.H. Rosenberg, and W.A. Walker. "When You Suspect Lactose Intolerance." *Patient Care* XIV(13):136, July, 1980.

Briggs, George M., and Doris Calloway. *Bogert's Nutrition and Physical Fitness.* Philadelphia: W.B. Saunders Co., 1979.

Cheraskin, E., W.M. Ringsdorf, and J.W. Clark. *Diet and Disease.* New Canaan, Conn.: Keats Publishing Co., 1968.

Fredericks, Carlton, and Herbert Bailey. *Food Facts and Fallacies.* New York: Galahad Books, 1965.

Fredericks, Carlton, and Herman Goodman, M.D. *Low Blood Sugar and You.* New York: Grosset & Dunlap, 1969.

Goodhart, R.S., and M.E. Shils. *Modern Nutrition in Health and Disease.* Philadelphia: Lea & Febiger, 1980.

Holt, L.E. *The Care and Feeding of Children.* New York: D. Appleton & Co., 1914.

————. *Food, Health and Growth.* New York: Macmillan, 1922.

Kugelmass, I. Newton. *Growing Superior Children.* Philadelphia: Appleton-Century, 1940.

————. *The Newer Nutrition in Pediatric Practice.* Philadelphia: Lippincott, 1946.

Levin, Simon S. *A Philosophy of Infant Feeding.* Springfield, Ill.: Charles C. Thomas, 1963.

Miller, J.J. *Nutrition and Tooth Decay.* West Chicago, Ill.: Miller Modalities, 1976.

Routh, C.H.F. *Infant Feeding and Its Influence on Life.* New York: William Wood & Co., 1879.

Sasaki, N. (1964) "The Relationship of Salt Intake to Hypertension in the Japanese." *Geriatrics* XIX:735, 1964.

Talking Food Company. Box 81, Charlestown, Ma.

Weimar Institute. *From the Weimar Kitchen.* Weimar, Ca., 1978.

Weimar, Michael. *The Skeptical Nutritionist.* New York: Macmillan, 1971.

———. *Weiner's Herbal.* New York: Stein & Day, 1980.

Williams, Roger J. *Nutrition Against Disease.* New York: Bantam Books, 1973.

Index

[315]

Recipe Index

ABOUT THE AUTHOR

Michael Weiner is the author of several books in the field of nutrition and herbalism, including *Earth Medicine—Earth Foods* and *The Skeptical Nutritionist.* After completing his study of human biology, he earned graduate degrees in ethnobotany and anthropology. Having worked with numerous folk healers in Fiji and Tonga in the South Pacific over a ten-year period, Mr. Weiner was awarded his doctorate in nutritional ethnomedicine from the University of California, Berkeley— the first degree of its kind. Currently the author maintains offices in San Francisco where he counsels individuals, corporations, and governmental officials in the use and misuse of herbs and nutrients.